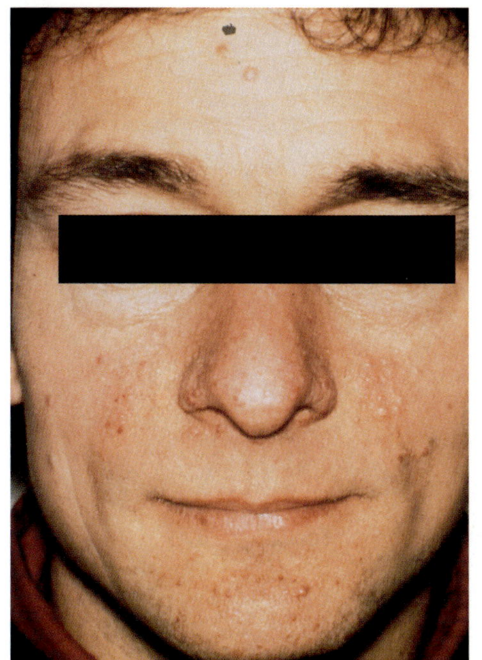

Slide 1

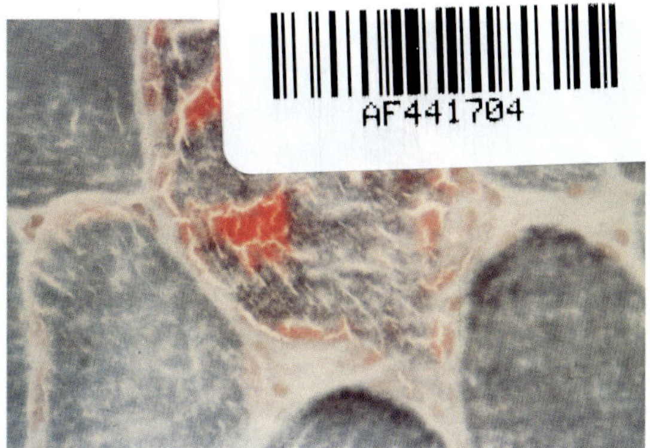

Slide 2

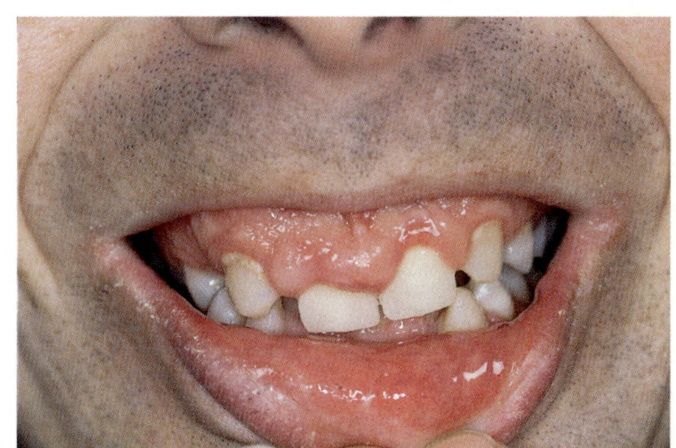

Slide 3

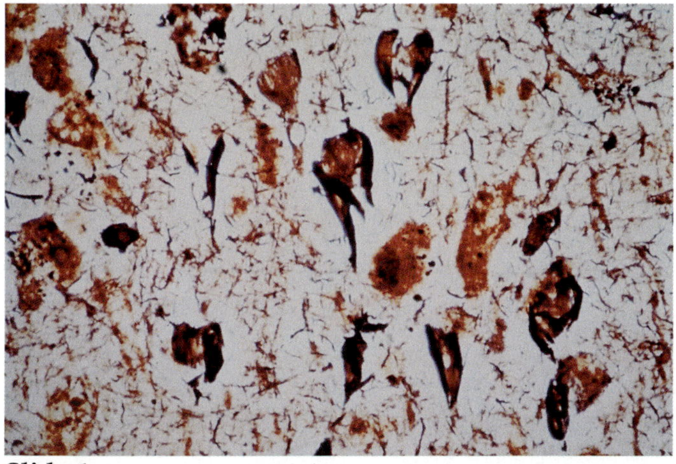

Slide 4

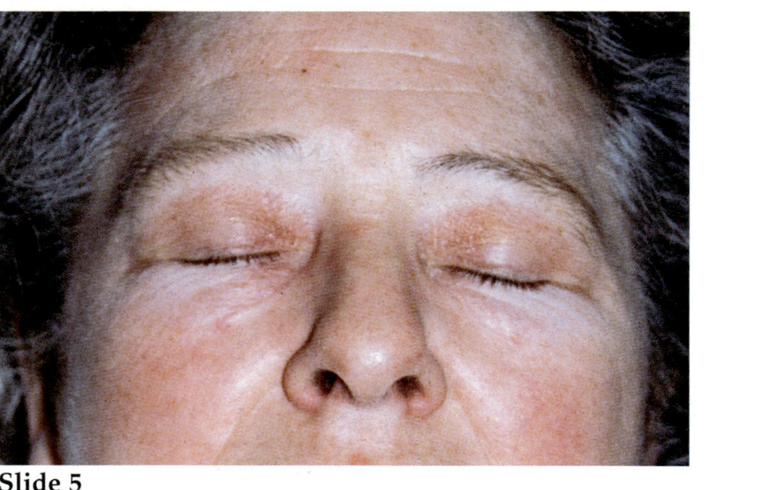

Slide 5

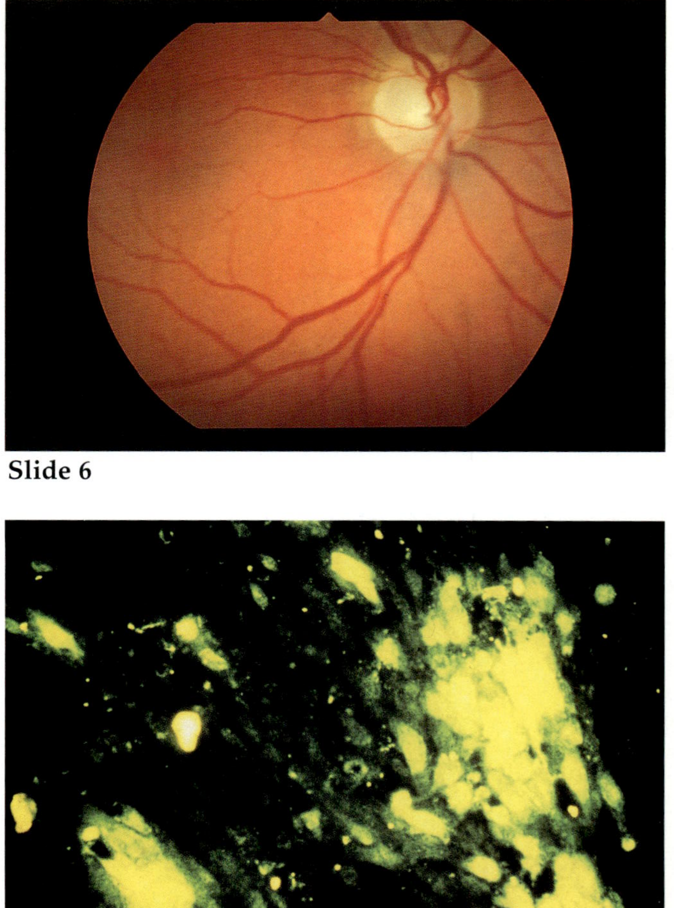

Slide 6

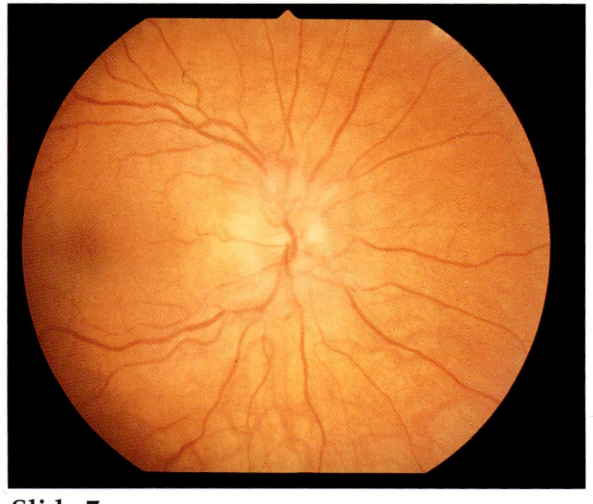

Slide 7

Slide 8

Neurology for the MRCP Part II

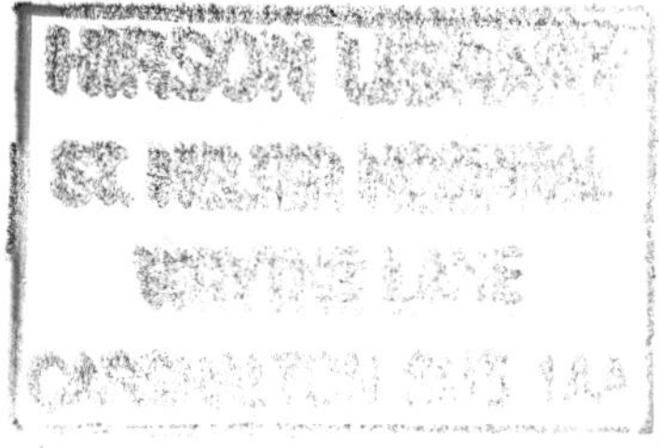

Neurology for the MRCP Part II

David Smith MD, MRCP
Consultant Neurologist, The Walton Centre for Neurology and Neurosurgery, Liverpool, UK

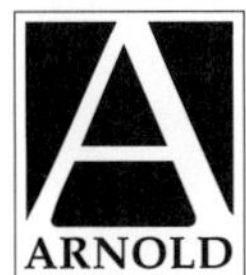

A member of the Hodder Headline Group
LONDON • SYDNEY • AUCKLAND
Co-published in the USA by
Oxford University Press, Inc., New York

First published in Great Britain 1998 by
Arnold, a member of the Hodder Headline group,
338 Euston Road, London NW1 3BH
http://www.arnoldpublishers.com

Co-published in the United States of America by
Oxford University Press, Inc.,
198 Madison Avenue, New York, NY 10016
Oxford is a registered trademark of Oxford University Press

Whilst the advice and information in this book is believed to be true and
accurate at the date of going to press, neither the author nor the publisher
can accept any legal responsibility or liability for any errors or omissions
that may be made. In particular (but without limiting the generality of the
preceding disclaimer) every effort has been made to check drug dosages;
however it is still possible that errors have been missed. Furthermore,
dosage schedules are constantly being revised and new side-effects
recognized. For these reasons the reader is strongly urged to consult the
drug companies' printed instructions before administering any of the drugs
recommended in this book.

British Library Cataloging in Publication Data
A catalogue record for this book is available from the British Library

Library of Congress Cataloguing-in-Publication Data
A catalog record for this book is available from the Library of Congress

ISBN 0 340 69175 1

Commissioning Editor: Georgina Bentliff
Project Editor: Melissa Morton
Production Editor: Liz Gooster
Production Controller: Rose James
Cover Design: Terry Griffiths

1 2 3 4 5 6 7 8 9 10

Typeset in 10/12 pt Palatino by J&L Composition Ltd, Filey, North Yorkshire
Printed and bound in Great Britain by JW Arrowsmith, Bristol

Contents

Preface

Neurological problems account for 20–25% of out-patient consultations and acute hospital admissions. Neurology, therefore, forms an important part of the MRCP examination.

Unfortunately, physicians in training often consider that neurology is complicated and view the subject with trepidation. This may be compounded by a tendency to concentrate on relatively rare conditions. Therefore, while I have included some 'small-print' cases, I have tried to focus attention on straightforward conditions and simple clinical lessons.

The majority of the grey cases are real patients. Some are too difficult for the MRCP, but detailed explanations are provided and some candidates might use these cases as opportunities for additional learning. When approaching these cases (as in clinical practice) ask three questions. First, does the pattern of symptoms and signs suggest an organic problem? Second, what is the anatomical site of the lesion(s)? Third, what is the underlying pathology? The latter is principally determined by the onset and course of symptoms.

With the exception of CSF, neurology does not easily lend itself to data interpretation. Therefore, several of the cases chosen reflect the effect of systemic conditions on the CNS. I have included five neurophysiology cases. These are not usually included in the MRCP, but interpretation of these tests is no more difficult than echocardiography or pulmonary function tests. Simple discussions of these techniques are included in the Neurology Section of *Medicine International*.

References are provided for the vivas only. For further reading I would strongly recommend Amminoff's *Neurology and General Medicine* (Churchill Livingstone, 2nd edition, 1995) while, for more detail, Adam's *Principles and Practice of Neurology* (McGraw Hill, 5th edition, 1995) is excellent.

I would like to acknowledge the contribution of my colleagues whose 'brains have been tapped', sometimes overtly, often surreptitiously, and my neuroradiological colleagues for their interpretations of the imaging. I would like to thank Parthenon Publishing for permission to reproduce the slides (2, 3, 4, 9, 16, 18, 22, 26, 39, 40) from Smith, DF, Appleton, RE, MacKenzie, JM and Chadwick, DW *An Atlas of Epilepsy* (Parthenon, New York, London, 1997). Thanks also to the Medical Photography Departments at Walton Hospital and Ysbyty Glan Clwyd for their reproductions, and to the patients for consenting to be photographed. Finally, thanks to my long-suffering secretary, Sue Brown, who typed the manuscript.

Normal Values

Haematology

White blood count	$4–11.0 \times 10^9/l$
Red blood count	$4.4–6.0 \times 10^{12}/l$
Haemoglobin	14–18 g/dl (male),
	12–16 g/dl (female)
Packed cell volume (PCV)	38.5–51 l/l
Mean cell volume (MCV)	80–100 fl
Mean cell haemoglobin (MCH)	27–33 pg
Mean cell haemoglobin concentration (MCHC)	32–37 g/dl
Platelets	$140–450 \times 10^9/l$
International normalized ratio (INR)	0.8–1.2
Activated partial thromboplastin time (APTT)	0.8–1.2
Serum B12	150–750 ng/l
Red cell folate	125–500 µg/l

Biochemistry

Sodium	136–144 mmol/l
Potassium	3.5–5.0 mmol/l
Urea	2.7–7.5 mmol/l
Creatinine	< 110 µmol/l
Glucose	Random
	3.6–8.4 mmol/l
	Fasting 3.6–5.5 mmol/l
Protein	60–80 g/l
Albumin	36–50 g/l
Alanine transferase (ALT)	11–55 IU/l
Aspartate transferase (AST)	13–42 IU/l
Gamma glutamyl transferase (GGT)	< 50 IU/l (male)
	< 30 IU/l (female)
Alkaline phosphatase	30–130 IU/l
Bilirubin	< 22 µmol/l
Calcium	2.18–2.62 mmol/l
Phosphate	0.7–1.6 mmol/l

Magnesium	0.6–1.10 mmol/l
Chloride	95–105 mmol/l
Creatine phosphokinase (CPK)	< 175 IU/l
T4	60–160 nmol/l
Free T4	10.3–25.8 pmol/l
Free T3	2.0–5.5 pmol/l
Thyroid stimulating hormone (TSH)	0.3–5.5 mU/l

Arterial blood gases

pH	7.36–7.42
pCO_2	35–45 mmHg
pO_2	90–100 mmHg
Base excess	+2.3 mmol/l
Standard bicarbonate	22–26 mmol/l

Cerebrospinal fluid

Red blood cells	< 5 /mm^3
White blood cells	< 5 /mm^3
Glucose	mmol/l (50–70% of blood level)
Protein	0.1–0.45 g/l

List of Abbreviations

ABN	Association of British Neurologists
ADEM	Acute disseminated encephalomyelitis
ADM	Abductor digiti minimi
ANCA	Antineutrophil cytoplasmic antibody
APB	Abductor pollicis brevis
AVM	Arterio-venous malformation
CD4 count	Number of T-helper cells
CIDP	Chronic inflammatory demyelinating polyneuropathy
CJD	Creutzfeldt–Jacob disease
CNS	Central nervous system
CSF	Cerebrospinal fluid
CT	Computed tomography
dsDNA	Double-stranded deoxyribose nucleic acid
DSM-IV	Diagnostic and Statistic Manual of Mental Disorders IV (American Psychiatric Association)
EBV	Epstein–Barr virus
ECG	Electrocardiogram
EDSS	Extended disability status scale
EEG	Electroencephalogram
EMG	Electromyogram
ESR	Erythrocyte sedimentation rate
FBC	Full blood count
FTA-abs	Fluorescent treponemal antibody
GBS	Guillain–Barré syndrome
GCSE	(1) General Certificate of Secondary Education (2) Generalized convulsive status elepticus
GSW	Generalized spike and wave
HbA$_1$C	Glycosylated haemoglobin
HbSAg	Hepatitis surface antigen
HIV	Human immunodeficiency virus
HLA	Human leucocyte antigen
HSV	*Herpes simplex* virus
HSV-DNA	*Herpes simplex* virus deoxyribose nucleic acid
HTLV-1	Human T-cell leukaemia virus-1
INO	Internuclear ophthalmoplegia
INR	International normalized ratio

IPD	Idiopathic Parkinson's disease
IQ	Intelligence quotient
LFT	Liver function test
MERRF	Myoclonic epilepsy with ragged red fibres
MND	Motor neurone disease
MR	Magnetic resonance
MRA	Magnetic resonance angiography
MRI	Magnetic resonance imaging
MS	Multiple sclerosis
NCS	Nerve conduction studies
NCV	Nerve conduction velocity
NHS	National Health Service
NR	Normal range
NSAIDs	Non-steroidal anti-inflammatory drugs
NTE	Neuropathy target esterase
PSGBS	Plasma Exchange Sandoglobulin in Guillain–Barré Study
PSVER	Pattern-shift visual evoked response
REM	Rapid eye movement
SLE	Systemic lupus erythematosus
TIA	Transient ischaemic attack
TPHA	*Treponema pallidium* haemagglutination
TS	Tuberous sclerosis
UTI	Urinary tract infection
VDRL	Venereal Diseases Research Laboratory
VER	Visual evoked response
VHL	Von Hippel–Landau
VMA	Vanillyl mandelic acid

Grey Cases

Question 1

One morning, a 54 year old man developed progressively worsening diplopia. Gait and speech were unaffected. After lunch he appeared to be sleeping but, 2 hours later, his wife found him to be unrousable.

On admission to hospital he was comatose with an obvious left third (III) nerve palsy and bilateral extensor plantar responses. Computed tomography (CT) scan, performed soon after arrival at hospital, and cerebrospinal fluid (CSF) were normal.

During the next week his conscious level fluctuated but improved sufficiently to permit a more formal examination which revealed a complete left III nerve palsy, a partial right III nerve palsy, dysarthria, weakness and ataxia of the right-sided limbs.

Where is the lesion?

Question 2

An 18 year old student had complained to the general practitioner about recurrent blackouts preceded by dizziness, buzzing in her ears and blurred vision. On regaining consciousness she was alway sweaty and sometimes vomited. On one occasion she had been incontinent of urine. Her friends reported that during the attacks she was usually quite pale and often exhibited brief twitching movements of her arms and legs.

Her general practitioner referred her to a specialist but, whilst waiting for an appointment, she was taken to casualty with a more severe attack. She had been found by her flatmate, slumped against the bathroom wall, pale and unrousable. She had been doubly incontinent and had bitten her tongue. She became lucid 30 minutes later when she recalled the usual warning symptoms prior to falling off the toilet seat.

Neurological and cardiac examination were normal.

(a) What was the cause of her admission to hospital?
(b) How should she be managed?

Answer 1

Left midbrain.

Comment

A magnetic resonance imaging (MRI) scan revealed an area of infarction on the left side of the midbrain. A number of eponymous syndromes cause an ipsilateral III nerve palsy with contralateral motor or sensory signs. These include: Weber's – III nerve palsy + hemiparesis; Claude's – III nervy palsy + tremor; Benedict's – III nerve palsy + hemianaesthesia + tremor. Because of the close anatomical association of the oculomotor nuclei, midbrain lesions commonly produce bilateral asymmetric III nerve palsies which are often associated with severely depressed consciousness owing to involvement of the ascending reticular pathways.

Answer 2

(a) Reflex anoxic seizure.
(b) Counselling about postural manoeuvres which can prevent loss of consciousness when the warning symptoms occur.

Comment

This is a common problem which is often misdiagnosed as epilepsy. The warning symptoms and the observed pallor and sweating are typical features of postural hypotension. The brief twitching movements are myoclonic jerks which commonly occur in simple faints. Furthermore, incontinence can occur in anyone who loses consciousness with a full bladder. Because she remained in an upright position after losing consciousness, the seizure was provoked by cerebral hypoxia. If the provocative factor has resolved, or can be avoided, provoked seizures do not carry an automatic driving ban.

Question 3

A 28 year old accountant had felt non-specifically unwell for 1 week. His symptoms included sore throat, mild headache, myalgia and lethargy. Despite this, he had continued to work but came home one morning because of worsening headache and a curious sensation in his right hand. At lunch he complained of 'difficulty finding the right word' and his wife found him to be somewhat confused. He went to bed and she phoned the general practitioner.

The general practitioner arrived within 1 hour to find him febrile and semi-comatose with a right hemiparesis. He had no neck stiffness or rash.

He was admitted to a local hospital where an urgent CT scan revealed diffuse low-density changes in the left hemisphere with patchy enhancement and mass effect. Immediately after the CT, he had a seizure complicated by a cardiorespiratory arrest necessitating ventilation. After discussion with the neurologist he was treated with intravenous antibiotics, acyclovir, mannitol and dexamethasone, and transferred to the neurosciences unit. He died soon after arrival without further investigations being performed. Consent for a postmortem was obtained.

Name two diagnostic possibilities.

Answer 3

Herpes simplex encephalitis.
Acute haemorrhagic leucoencephalitis, the most severe form of acute disseminated encephalomyelitis (ADEM).

Comment

These two conditions are clinically indistinguishable. They may produce a remarkably insidious prodromal (flu-like) illness followed by a devastating acute phase. CSF usually reveals raised protein, pleomorphic leucocytosis and high red cell count. Death may occur within hours of the first neurological symptoms despite aggressive treatment. Whilst acyclovir is of proven benefit in herpes simplex encephalitis, this condition still carries a mortality rate of 20–30%. Traditionally, steroids have been used in patients with ADEM but there is no controlled evidence of efficacy. Herpes simplex encephalitis can be reliably diagnosed within 24 hours using the polymerase chain reaction for detection of specific *Herpes simplex* virus deoxyribose nucleic acid (HSV-DNA). Whilst the MRI may reveal large plaques of demyelination in milder forms of ADEM, in the most severe forms the haemorrhagic features predominate and demyelination may be insignificant. Consequently, the MRI may be non-specifically abnormal.

Question 4

A 45 year old lady gave a 5-year history of progressive leg weakness and urgency of micturition. She had experienced an episode of right mid-thoracic herpes zoster prior to the onset of these neurological symptoms, but was unsure of the precise temporal relationship between the shingles and her presenting problem. She also reported a single episode of acute lumbago, not associated with radicular pain, 15 years previously. She specifically denied other neurological episodes.

Family history was non-contributory. She admits to being a heavy smoker but had no systemic complaints.

General examination was normal. Examination of the nervous system revealed spastic monoparesis of the left leg and weakness of hip flexion on the right. Knee reflexes were obtained with reinforcement, ankle jerks were absent but plantar responses were extensor. There was patchy diminution of pain and temperature sensation from L3–S1 on the left and L2–3 on the right. Joint position sense was normal. Upper limbs and cranial limbs were normal.

The following investigations were normal or negative: full blood count (FBC), erythrocyte sedimentation rate (ESR), biochemical profile, Venereal Diseases Research Laboratory (VDRL) and *Treponema pallidum* haemagglutination (TPHA). Lower limb nerve conduction studies revealed no evidence of a peripheral neuropathy.

(a) Where is the lesion?
(b) Name three possible causes.

Answer 4

(a) Conus medullaris.
(b) Benign tumour (meningioma, ependymoma).
     Spinal dural arteriovenous malformation.
     Demyelination.

Comment

The clinical signs (patchy lower limb motor and sensory deficit, early bladder involvement, absent ankle jerks and extensor plantar responses) indicate a conus lesion. MRI of lumbar and thoracic spine revealed no intrinsic lesion and a normal myelogram effectively excludes an arteriovenous malformation (AVM). An MRI of brain revealed a few periventicular lesions and immuno-fixation of CSF was positive for oligoclonal bands. While a definite diagnosis has not been established, the investigations suggest demyelination and the likeliest diagnosis is primary progressive multiple sclerosis (MS).

Question 5

A 63 year old housewife had a 2-month history of depressive symptoms which, not unreasonably, had been attributed to the recent death of her brother. However, during the next 2 weeks, she became 'blind' and, because no ocular cause could be identified, she was referred to a psychiatrist. Her husband had also observed that she had lost the ability to locate objects, or even his voice, in space. After admission to hospital her conscious level deteriorated and she was transferred to a neurology ward.

She was afebrile with no neck stiffness. She was semi-comatose: groaning, opening her eyes to speech and localizing pain. She appeared to be blind, but pupillary reactions and fundoscopy were normal. Limited cranial nerve examination was normal, she had no involuntary movements and, apart from symmetrically brisk flexes, there were no limb signs.

The following tests were normal or negative: full blood count, biochemical profile, thyroid function, antinuclear factor, immunoglobulin levels, CSF and CT of brain.

Within 2 weeks she became deeply comatose with rigidity of all four limbs, paratonia and frequent myoclonic jerks. The likely diagnosis and prognosis was discussed with her family who agreed that further intervention was not justified. She died of pneumonia and a postmortem was performed.

(a) What is the diagnosis?
(b) Name one useful non-invasive investigation.

Answer 5

(a) Creutzfeldt–Jacob disease.
(b) EEG.

Comment

The history of rapidly progressive dementia, often with psychiatric symptoms initially, cortical blindness, spatial disorientation, myoclonus and rigidity culminating in death is typical of Creutzfeldt–Jacob disease (CJD). An electroencephalogram (EEG) performed early in the illness may be unremarkable but, as the disease progresses, repeat EEGs reveal generalized periodic sharp wave discharges most evident during periods of arousal. CJD is an infectious condition and the transmissible agent is now known to be a prion protein. Specific procedures, for example, corneal grafts and human growth hormone injections, have been implicated but, in most cases, the cause cannot be identified.

Question 6

A 50 year old policeman was referred because of 'intractable migraine'. He gave a 2-year history of daily episodes of left temporal and periorbital pain sometimes associated with drooping of the eyelid, redness of the eye and rhinorrhoea. Each episode lasted 20–30 minutes but these tended to recur 6–10 times per day. His symptoms had not responded to adequate trials of three different prophylactic agents: pizotifen, propranolol and amitriptyline. He had tried analgesics but was aware that his symptoms resolved before the tablets were absorbed.

There is no relevant past medical or family history, neurological examination is normal and, apart from thickening of the maxillary antra, CT of head is normal.

(a) Name two possible diagnoses and state which is most likely.
(b) What is the treatment?

Answer 6

(a) Chronic paroxysmal hemicrania.
     Cluster headache (migrainous neuralgia).
(b) Indomethacin.

Comment

Apart from a unilateral headache, this man has no other features of classical migraine: visual aura, nausea and vomiting, positive family history.

Chronic paroxysmal hemicrania and cluster headache have several common features: location of pain, duration of attacks, associated sympathetic features. However, whilst clusters may last for months it would be most unusual for a single cluster to persist for 2 years. Recognition of chronic paroxysmal hemicrania is important because, although it is uncommon, most patients respond dramatically to indomethacin.

Question 7

Ten days after a flu-like illness, a 36 year old shop assistant developed 'pins and needles in her legs'. Within 48 hours the sensory disturbance had spread to her abdomen, her legs were weak and she had difficulty passing urine.

On admission she was in acute urinary retention. She had a mild spastic paraparesis, a mid-thoracic spinothalamic sensory level and a slightly ataxic gait.

An MRI scan revealed high signal lesions in the thoracic and cervical cord. CSF protein was elevated but there were no cells. She was catheterized and received five boluses of intravenous methylprednisolone. Within 1 week bladder sensation had recovered permitting successful removal of the catheter, her gait had improved and she was allowed home.

Two weeks later, whilst her mobility had virtually recovered, she developed painful loss of vision of the left eye. Visual acuity was limited to counting fingers, the optic disc was blurred and there was a relative afferent pupillary defect. Three days later, without treatment, her vision was improving but she had a large centrocaecal scotoma. Visual evoked responses were performed: left 178 ms, right 105 ms. MRI of brain revealed a few high-intensity lesions in the cerebral hemispheres and cerebellar peduncles. Immunofixation of CSF, from the first admission, was negative for oligoclonal bands. Viral serology confirmed a recent influenza B infection (titre 1:640).

What is the differential diagnosis?

Answer 7

Multiple sclerosis.
Postinfective demyelination.

Comment

Whilst there is clinical and investigative evidence of demyelinating lesions in the cerebral nervous system (CNS) which are separated in space (spinal cord, optic nerve) and time, the 'obvious diagnosis' of multiple sclerosis (MS) is by no means secure. Alternatively, it could be argued that this is a monophasic illness which followed a scrologically confirmed viral infection. Some authorities assert that, in this situation, MS cannot be diagnosed with confidence unless new, gadolinium-enhancing lesions are seen on MRI scan 1 year after the initial symptoms.

Question 8

A 52 year old hotelier was referred because of fasciculations in his upper limbs. He denied weakness or bulbar symptoms, but complained of insomnia, memory problems and word-finding difficulties.

Examination revealed disinhibition, impaired verbal fluency, mild expressive dysphasia and impaired short-term memory. Cranial nerves were normal. He had fasciculations affecting the shoulder girdle muscles, biceps and triceps bilaterally, but no wasting or weakness. Reflexes were symmetrically brisk with flexor plantar responses. There were no sensory signs.

An EMG revealed evidence of chronic active denervation in the muscles sampled from all four limbs. The following tests were normal or negative: FBC, ESR, biochemical profile, thyroid function, serum B12 and red cell folate, antinuclear factor, syphilis serology, CSF, MRI of the brain and EEG. Neuropsychological assessment revealed diminished insight and pronounced cognitive impairment with a significant decline in full-scale intelligence quotient (IQ), impairments in short-term memory for visual and verbal material, and striking deficits on tests of frontal lobe function.

What is the diagnosis?

Answer 8

Motor neurone disease (MND) with frontal lobe dementia.

Comment

Despite the absence of weakness and wasting, the combination of visible fasciculations and chronic active denervation on electromyogram (EMG) is diagnostic of an anterior horn cell disorder (MND). Contrary to previously held beliefs, cognitive problems do occur in patients with MND. These are clinically significant in 5%, while subtle deficits, detected by neuropsychological testing only, occur in 25% of cases. However, the prominence of cognitive symptoms in the presence of preserved motor function is unusual.

Question 9

The parents of a 16 year old schoolgirl had noticed that she was sometimes 'twitchy', particularly at breakfast times. This was most likely if she was tired or menstruating. Initially these episodes were thought to be behavioural but, 6 months later, on the morning after a late-night party, she had a witnessed convulsion without warning. There was no relevant past medical or family history, and examination was normal.

She was referred to a local physician who arranged an EEG which was reported as being consistent with 'grand mal epilepsy'. Therefore, phenytoin was prescribed but she reported monthly convulsions despite increasing doses of phenytoin and the addition of carbamazepine.

(a) What is the diagnosis?
(b) What treatment is appropriate?

Answer 9

(a) Juvenile myoclonic epilepsy.
(b) Sodium valproate.

Comment

Epilepsy syndromes are defined by the age of seizure onset, seizure type(s), EEG characteristics and concomitant clinical features. They are useful in terms of defining aetiology/need for investigation, predicting prognosis and selecting treatment.

Juvenile myoclonic epilepsy commences between the ages of 8 and 26 in neurologically intact individuals. Seizure types include myoclonic jerks, tonic–clonic seizures and, sometimes, absences, which usually occur within 2 hours of wakening and which are precipitated by sleep deprivation, alcohol and menstruation. The characteristic EEG abnormality is a 4–6 Hz generalized spike and wave, but it can be normal or, indeed, show a combination of focal and generalized epileptiform discharges. Although a positive family history is present in only 30–40% of cases, this condition is genetically determined and has been linked to the short arm of chromosome 6. Approximately 80% of patients are rendered seizure-free on sodium valproate. However, most, if not all, relapse if treatment is withdrawn and, therefore, lifelong treatment is recommended.

This syndrome is important for several reasons:

- It is the commonest of the idiopathic generalized epilepsies, accounting for 5–8% of all epilepsy;
- Patients present to paediatricians, adult physicians and neurologists;
- Failure to recognize the condition is common, resulting in ineffective treatment with carbamazepine or ill-advised cessation of treatment in patients who become seizure-free on sodium valproate.

Question 10

A 53 year old company director gave a 12-month history of progressive painless left foot drop. This was aggravated by exercise and, during the previous 3 months, he had noted a tendency to trip. He also complained of minimal weakness of pincer grip in the right hand. He had no other neurological symptoms.

General examination was normal. Cranial nerves and upper limbs were also normal. There was wasting of the intrinsic muscles of the left foot, reduced tone at the ankle, weakness of dorsiflexion, inversion, eversion and plantar flexion and a diminished left ankle jerk. All other reflexes were easily obtained and plantar responses were flexor. There were no sensory signs.

The following investigations were normal or negative: FBC, ESR, biochemistry, immunoglobulins, serum B12 and red cell folate, syphilis serology, CSF, MRI of lumbar spine and whole spine myelogram. An EMG was inconclusive: the main finding was evidence of active denervation in the muscles supplied by both the peroneal and tibial nerves.

(a) What is the most likely diagnosis?
(b) How might this be established?

Answer 10

(a) Motor neurone disease.
(b) Follow-up and repeat EMG.

Comment

There are several possible explanations for a unilateral foot drop. Whilst the patient reports fatiguability, it is very unusual for myasthenia gravis to present with lower limb symptoms only and there was no EMG evidence to support this diagnosis. The distribution of weakness and absence of sensory symptoms or pain militate strongly against a single peripheral nerve or root lesion. Other causes of fatiguable weakness include spinal cord AVM and lumbar canal stenosis, but these are excluded by the normal myelogram and MRI, respectively. Finally, there are no lateralized pyramidal signs to suggest a central cause.

Apart from the exclusion of the other possibilities, the focal onset of purely motor symptoms (wasting and weakness) and EMG evidence of denervation is highly suggestive of anterior horn cell disease and the rate of progression favours motor neurone disease rather than late-onset spinal muscular atrophy. At follow-up, 3 months later, weakness of pincer grip in the right hand was clinically evident and repeat EMG revealed chronic active denervation in all four limbs.

Question 11

A 73 year old retired miner was referred with a 6-year history of involuntary movements which, while constant, had improved with tetrabenazine. It was thought that his verbal aggression, considered to be the consequence of his physical problems, had also improved with the treatment of the movement disorder. He remained self-caring and interested in current affairs and sport on television.

Apart from pneumoconiosis, his medical history was unremarkable. Specifically, he had no history of cerebral insult, no vascular risk factors, no systemic complaints and he was taking no other medication. There was no family history of neurological disease.

Blood pressure 160/95. He had generalized choreiform movements. Otherwise, neurological and systematic examination were normal.

The following tests were normal/negative: full blood count, ESR, anti-nuclear factor and autoantibody screen, sodium, potassium, glucose, calcium, magnesium, renal and liver function tests, and serological tests for syphilis. MRI, under general anaesthetic, revealed age-related atrophy and no focal pathology.

(a) What condition should be excluded?
(b) Why?

Answer 11

(a) Late-onset Huntington's disease.
(b) Autosomal dominant inheritance (with anticipation).

Comment

Late-onset chorea can be hereditary or symptomatic of a wide range of systemic/cerebral pathologies. Iatrogenic (drug-induced) chorea is probably commonest but this man was taking no medication. Metabolic, immunological and relevant infective (neurosyphilis) conditions have been excluded. Atheromatous cerebrovascular disease is a rare cause of chorea and, given his normal blood pressure and the magnetic resonance (MR) appearances, diffuse small-vessel disease affecting the basal ganglia seems unlikely. The temptation to label this as 'senile chorea' should be resisted; some authorities doubt the existence of such a condition.

DNA testing revealed that this man had Huntington's disease. This condition is characterized by a triad of dominant inheritance, choreoathetosis and progressive dementia. The responsible genetic defect is a trinucleotide expansion on the short arm of chromosome 4. While onset is commonest in mid-life, presentation in the seventh or eighth decades is well-recognized and, in late-onset cases, the movement disorder may predominate while cognitive/behavioural features remain relatively mild. Recognition is important because, apart from dominant inheritance, Huntington's disease displays the phenomenon of anticipation in males, i.e. earlier age of onset in successive generations.

Question 12

A 72 year old woman gave a 20-year history of very gradually progressive gait difficulty. She was initially aware of slight unsteadiness whilst ballroom dancing but was able to continue dancing for many years. During the last 2 years her symptoms had progressed more rapidly, she reported a few falls and had adopted a wide-based gait. More recently, she had noticed difficulty focusing especially when going downstairs.

Her physical appearance was normal. She walked with a broad-based, ataxic gait and had mild heel-shin ataxia. She had horizontal nystagmus on lateral gaze and prominent down-beat nystagmus on down gaze. There were no other cranial nerve or limb signs.

Where is the lesion?

Question 13

A 62 year old man presented with a tremor of his right hand. Examination revealed a resting tremor, cog-wheel rigidity at the right wrist and loss of right arm swing whilst walking. A diagnosis of idiopathic Parkinson's disease was made but, because he had no functional disability, treatment was not commenced.

Six months later his symptoms had progressed and, therefore, Sinemet was started. Over the next 3 years, his condition steadily deteriorated despite increasing doses of Sinemet and the addition of bromocriptine.

He had no history of head trauma, vascular disease or exposure to psychotropic drugs. He specifically denied cognitive or psychiatric symptoms, sphincter disturbance or postural dizziness.

When referred for a second opinion, examination revealed expressionless facies, low-volume speech and moderately severe, asymmetric (right more than left) extrapyramidal signs. There were no cognitive, pyramidal or cerebellar signs, and his blood pressure was normal.

What is the likeliest diagnosis?

Answer 12

Cervico-medullary junction or foramen magnum.

Comment

Down-beat nystagmus is a classical localizing sign. Specific causes include bony abnormalities (platybasia or basilar impression), syringobulbia, foramen magnum tumours and, particularly, Chiari malformations. Bony abnormalities in this region are usually associated with physical signs, notably a short neck. The patient had no bulbar symptoms. Furthermore, whilst foramen magnum tumours are usually benign, extramedullary lesions, they typically cause local pain and progression over 1–2 years to a spastic tetraparesis.

This patient's MRI scan revealed a type 1 Chiari malformation (extension of the cerebellar tonsils and medulla into the cervical canal without meningomyelocele). In most cases these present in childhood but a significant proportion do not manifest themselves until adult life. Presentations include raised intracranial pressure, progressive cerebellar ataxia, syringomyelia or a combination thereof. Treatment depends on the degree of disability. In this case, because of progressive ataxia, she underwent cervical laminectomy and decompression of the foramen magnum.

Answer 13

Striato-nigral degeneration.

Comment

This patient presents with classical features of idiopathic Parkinson's disease (IPD). However, one of the important diagnostic criteria is a dramatic (70–100%) initial response to therapy. There are several other conditions with prominent extrapyramidal features which do not respond to dopamine replacement therapy, but, unlike this patient, these conditions are associated with clinical features which indicate more widespread neurodegenerative disease. About 10–15% of patients with 'typical IPD' do not respond to treatment. The majority of these individuals have striato-nigral degeneration.

Question 14

A 75 year old woman gave a 4-month history of progressive sensory symptoms in her right hand and distal forearm and weakness of right hand grip. Ten years previously she had a lumpectomy and radiotherapy for a right breast carcinoma. Six years later she had a mastectomy and, subsequently, removal of a local recurrence.

She was systematically well, but had weakness of all intrinsic muscles of the right hand, finger flexion and extension and wrist flexion. The right supinator jerk was absent. She had impaired cutaneous perception to pin prick affecting C6, 7 and 8 dermatomes.

Nerve conduction studies revealed a brachial plexopathy predominantly affecting the lower and middle trunks. CSF, including cytocentrifuge for malignant cells, was normal.

(a) Name two possible causes for this presentation.
(b) How might these be differentiated?

Question 15

A 57 year old builder presented to casualty with a sudden onset of painless double vision. His past medical history included cervical and lumbar spondylosis, late-onset, diet-controlled diabetes mellitus and episodes of renal colic. He smokes 20 cigarettes daily but consumes no alcohol.

His blood pressure was 176/104 but his cardiovascular system was otherwise normal. Ocular examination revealed a mild left ptosis and a mild left-divergent squint with impairment of adduction and elevation of the eye. Pupillary reactions were normal. He had symmetrically brisk reflexes with an extensor right plantar response but no significant motor or sensory deficits.

Random blood sugar was 9.8 mmol/l with a glycosylated haemoglobin (HbA_1C) of 8.9%. Otherwise, haematology and biochemistry were normal. A routine CT scan of the brain was also normal.

(a) What is the most likely explanation for this presentation?
(b) Name three aspects of treatment.

Answer 14

(a) Malignant infiltration of the brachial plexus.
     Radiation-induced brachial plexopathy.
(b) Surgical exploration and biopsy of brachial plexus.

Comment

These two possibilities are difficult to distinguish on clinical grounds. Furthermore, both conditions are progressive but carry different prognoses for survival. In statistical terms, involvement of the lower and middle trunks is more likely to be due to malignant infiltration. MR images of the brachial plexus are rarely of significant quality to distinguish between these two possibilities and, therefore, surgical exploration is the only method of reliably establishing the diagnosis.

Answer 15

(a) Intrinsic third nerve palsy.
(b) Treat the hypertension, treat the diabetes mellitus and start aspirin.

Comment

The sudden onset of a painless, pupil-sparing, partial third nerve palsy in a middle-aged man with three risk factors for atherosclerosis is most likely to be due to an intrinsic lesion. The presumed mechanism is atherosclerotic/embolic occlusion of the vasa nervosum. Management should concentrate on treatment of vascular risk factors. Most patients recover fully within a few months.

A small proportion of extrinsic lesions present in this manner. A high-dose contrast-enhanced CT, with thin cuts through the orbits, will detect the vast majority of posterior communicating artery aneurysms. However, up to 4% of all 'extrinsic' third nerve palsies are due to basilar or superior cerebellar artery aneurysms. Until recently, absolute exclusion of such lesions required four-vessel angiography but the advent of magnetic resonance angiography (MRA) provides a non-invasive method of visualizing the intracranial circulation.

Question 16

A 67 year old man presented with a gradually progressive gait disturbance, apathy and difficulty recognizing familiar faces. He reported urinary frequency and nocturia, but no incontinence. He had no history of cerebral insult and, apart from well-controlled hypertension, he had no vascular risk factors.

Examination of the fundi and cranial nerves was normal. He had an apraxic gait with no motor or sensory deficit in the limbs.

Formal neuropsychological examination revealed no evidence of generalized intellectual decline but there was impairment of recognition memory, attention, verbal fluency and higher executive functions. Definitive investigation and treatment occurred and he made a full recovery.

What is the most likely diagnosis?

Answer 16

Intermittent (normal) pressure hydrocephalus.

Comment

The term 'normal pressure hydrocephalus' is misleading. There is, in fact, intermittent elevation of intraventricular pressure which produces characteristic appearances on imaging: periventricular lucency, representing leakage of CSF into surrounding tissues, without cerebral atrophy or diffuse white matter ischaemia.

In approximately 50% of cases there is a history of significant head trauma, meningeal disease (subarachnoid haemorrhage, meningitis) or a tumour obstructing the CSF pathways. In the remaining 50% the condition is idiopathic. The classical triad of ataxia, dementia and incontinence is also incorrect. The true picture is that of gait apraxia and frontal lobe dysfunction, without dementia, while incontinence is an inconsistent feature.

Investigation should include MRI to exclude diffuse white matter ischaemia and CSF examination for evidence of meningeal disease.

In carefully selected cases, ventriculoperitoneal shunting can be dramatically effective. However, this form of treatment was brought into disrepute because patients with diffuse cerebrovascular disease, probably Bingswanger's encephalopathy, were inappropriately treated. Not only do these patients fail to improve but shunting is often complicated by subdural haematomata.

Question 17

A 35 year old farmer developed a mild illness comprising of running eyes, urinary frequency and diarrhoea which resolved within 48 hours. One week later he developed painful cramps in his calves and 'pins and needles' in his hands and feet. Two days later he was admitted to hospital because of progressive difficulty with walking.

Examination of cranial nerves was normal. He had mild weakness of intrinsic hand muscles and a severe bilateral foot drop. Supinator and ankle reflexes were absent, but all other reflexes were obtainable. There was a 'glove and stocking' sensory loss with a marked proprioceptive deficit in his feet.

Nerve conduction studies revealed a severe, distal axonal motor and sensory neuropathy with mildly delayed nerve conduction velocities.

He was thought to have an unusual axonal variant of Guillain–Barré syndrome and, therefore, received a 5-day course of intravenous immuno-globulin. During the next 3–4 weeks his neuropathy partially recovered, but repeat examinations reveal lower limb spasticity and a persisting sensory ataxia.

(a) What is the diagnosis?
(b) What treatment might have influenced the outcome?

Answer 17

(a) Organophosphate neuropathy.
(b) None.

Comment

A history of subacute neuropathy preceded by a diarrhoeal illness does suggest acute Guillain–Barré syndrome. Furthermore, an axonal variant is well recognized. However, the preservation of reflexes and the prominent sensory signs, confirmed electrophysiologically, strongly mitigate against this diagnosis.

His occupation suggests that he may have been exposed to neurotoxic insecticides or pesticides of which the most common are the organophosphates. His initial symptoms represent mild cholinergic overactivity. Organophosphates which inhibit neuropathy target esterase (NTE) cause a severe distal axonal neuropathy within 1–3 weeks of exposure. The peripheral neurotoxicity is self-limiting but outcome is directly related to the severity of the neuropathy at the nadir of the illness. Furthermore, as the neuropathy recovers, signs of spinal cord toxicity are unmasked. These are permanent and there is no effective treatment.

Question 18

A 27 year old single man was referred to a specialist for management of his epilepsy. He was the product of a full-term normal delivery and reached normal motor milestones. At the age of 18 months, he had a prolonged febrile convulsion with a postictal right hemiparesis which recovered fully.

His non-febrile seizures started at the age of 6. A typical attack is preceded by rising epigastric sensation and an olfactory hallucination. He is observed to stare and exhibit oral automatisms. He reports occasional secondary generalized tonic–clonic seizures. He has had no significant remission despite trials of all available antiepileptic drugs. Despite achieving seven GCSE passes, he has never obtained gainful employment.

Examination reveals slight underdevelopment of the right lower face. EEGs have been non-specifically abnormal or have shown a left temporal sharp wave focus. CT scans have been normal.

(a) What is the pathological diagnosis?
(b) What is the most appropriate treatment?

Answer 18

(a) Ammon's horn or mesial temporal sclerosis.
(b) Temporal lobectomy.

Comment

This man has classical complex partial seizures of medial temporal (hippocampal) origin. Some features (postictal hemiparesis, underdevelopment of the right lower face) suggest left hemisphere pathology.

The history of a complex early febrile convulsion and subsequent development of refractory temporal lobe epilepsy is highly suggestive of Ammon's horn sclerosis, which, pathologically, involves a characteristic pattern of hippocampal neuronal loss and gliosis. CT scans are usually normal but the associated hippocampal atrophy is readily detected by MRI. Subtle degrees of atrophy are detectable by MRI with measurement of hippocampal volumes.

In patients with long-standing epilepsy, manipulation of drug therapy is extremely unlikely to produce sustained remission. In contrast, if presurgical evaluation is satisfactory, temporal lobe resection carries a 70% chance of prolonged remission and, consequently, a realistic chance of employment.

Question 19

A 34 year old woman noticed numbness of the left axilla, medial aspect of the left arm and hand. Over the next 4 months the sensory deficit extended to involve the whole arm and shoulder, and the anterior and posterior aspects of the left side of her chest. She volunteered impairment of temperature sensation in the same distribution. She denied lower limb or sphincter symptoms.

Past medical history was unremarkable but she had sustained a 'whiplash injury' in a road traffic accident 2 years previously.

Cranial nerves were normal. She had loss of pin prick and temperature sensation in a 'hemicape' distribution over the left chest and arm. Light touch, joint position and vibration sense were normal. Apart from slight thinning of the intrinsic muscles of the left hand, there were no motor deficits.

(a) State two pathologies, in order of likelihood, which could explain this presentation.
(b) What investigation is indicated?

Question 20

A 21 year old student was referred because of blackouts. On closer questioning it transpired that these were preceded by symptoms which evolved in a fairly stereotyped manner. These involved blurred vision with patchy loss of vision in both visual fields, followed by dizziness, peripheral paraesthesia, unsteadiness and slurred speech. After 10–15 minutes her symptoms may resolve spontaneously or progress to a severe occipital headache at which time she would 'blackout'. Her friends observed pallor and sweating, but there were no convulsive features.

What is the diagnosis?

Answer 19

(a) Syringomyelia
Demyelination.
(b) MRI of cervical and thoracic spine.

Comment

This woman has a segmental (suspended), dissociated sensory deficit which can only be caused by a long, intrinsic cord lesion. Given the progressive course of her symptoms, a syrinx is much more likely than demyelination.

The clinical presentation of syringomyelia varies according to the associated features and the extent of the syrinx. Type 1 syringomyelia, which accounts for approximately 90% of cases, is associated with the obstruction of the foramen magnum, usually by a type 1 Chiari malformation. The idiopathic variety (type 2) is not associated with foramen magnum obstruction. Type 3 occurs in conjunction with other diseases of the cord, notably traumatic necrosis, intramedullary tumours and arachnoiditis.

The initial presentation usually involves segmental atrophy and loss of reflexes in the upper limbs and segmental, dissociated sensory loss in the upper limbs. However, the absence of motor features, whilst rare, is well documented. The course is highly variable but progression to a spastic ataxic paraparesis usually occurs.

In this case, the history of trauma is not relevant. The MRI revealed a syrinx extending from C3 to T6 and a type 1 Chiari malformation.

Answer 20

Vertebrobasilar migraine.

Comment

The bilateral visual symptoms, ataxia and dysarthria indicate a disturbance of the posterior circulation and the gradual evolution of symptoms (plus headache) typifies migraine as opposed to transient ischaemic attacks. Whilst the peripheral sensory symptoms might suggest hyperventilation, the rest of the clinical picture is clearly organic. Reflex syncope, induced by pain, is a common feature of this condition.

Question 21

A 67 year old man presented to casualty with a rapid onset of leg weakness. The admitting doctor noticed left facial weakness and left leg weakness, but he recorded no other neurological signs. Thinking the problem was cerebral, he ordered a CT scan which was normal.

The following day, repeat examination revealed global weakness of the left leg, mild proximal weakness of the right leg, absent lower limb reflexes and impaired touch sensation in both legs. He had to be catheterized because of painless retention of urine. A normal MRI of the spine excluded extrinsic cord compression. Because of the 'lower motor neurone signs', he was referred to a neurologist with a putative diagnosis of atypical Guillain–Barré syndrome.

His only medical history of note was hypertension for which he was taking nifedipine.

Examination revealed a flaccid, areflexic, asymmetric (left worst than right) paraplegia with loss of pain and temperature sensation below T8 but normal joint position sense. Upper limbs and cranial nerves were normal.

What is the diagnosis?

Answer 21

Spinal cord infarction (anterior spinal artery thrombosis).

Comment

There was some confusion over the anatomical localization of the lesion. Firstly, the left facial weakness had not been volunteered by the patient and, on questioning his wife, it transpired that the facial asymmetry was longstanding!

When the sphincter disturbance was noted, a spinal cause was considered but not excluded by the normal MRI. While flaccidity and areflexia suggest a lower motor neurone problem, it is important to recognize that these are features of 'spinal shock', a common consequence of trauma or ischaemia.

The blood supply to the spinal cord involves a paired series of segmental arteries arising from the aorta, and branches of the subclavian and internal iliac arteries. The upper middle and lower reticulomedullary arteries unite to form the anterior median spinal artery which lies in the anterior sulcus of the cord. Perforating branches supply the ventral two-thirds of the cord including the ventral grey matter, and the corticospinal and spinothalamic tracts.

Infarction of the cord is usually the result of disease of the large medullary arteries or the aorta. This produces a typical constellation of signs: motor paralysis, loss of spinothalamic sensation below the level of the lesion, sparing of proprioception and loss of sphincter function. Initially, there is 'spinal shock' but typical upper motor neurone signs evolve over a period of a few weeks. Prognosis for recovery of motor function is poor but bladder function may improve unless infarction involves the sacral segments of the cord.

Question 22

A 35 year old woman suddenly experienced distortion of vision. Initially, she was aware of flickering lines within both visual fields. When this symptom resolved, she described a right hemianopic field defect which persisted for 30 minutes. Later that day, she developed a mild generalized headache and neck stiffness which persisted for approximately a week.

Apart from hypertension during pregnancy, she had no past medical history of note. She did not smoke and there was no family history of migraine. General cardiac and neurological examination were entirely normal.

The following investigations were normal or negative: FBC, ESR, glucose, cholesterol, lupus anticoagulant, anticardiolipin antibody, antinuclear factor and serological tests for syphilis. A non-invasive diagnostic test was performed.

(a) What is the diagnosis?
(b) What was the diagnostic test?

Answer 22

(a) Right vertebral artery dissection.
(b) T_1-weighted axial MRI scan of neck.

Comment

Whilst the gradual evolution of visual symptoms might suggest a migrainous attack, the subsequent development of a persistent, non-specific headache and neck stiffness makes this diagnosis unlikely. Clinically, therefore, this should be labelled as a vertebrobasilar transient ischaemic attack in a young person with negative vascular investigations. Extracranial vertebral artery dissection is a well-recognized cause of this presentation and, if there is a history of trauma, this is often trivial.

This diagnosis is confirmed by the identification of blood in the arterial wall on axial T_1-weighted MRI of the neck and disturbed blood flow within the vertebral artery demonstrated by MRA. With the wider availability of these non-invasive investigations, this condition should always be excluded in a young person presenting with a vertebrobasilar transient ischaemic attack (TIA).

The natural history of these lesions has not been defined and, at present, treatment with aspirin should be continued for 6 months, with warfarin reserved for patients having further TIAs despite aspirin.

Question 23

A 20 year old student presented with a 4-year history of episodes in which she is unable to stop herself from falling asleep. These events occur in situations where drowsiness might be expected but also in completely inappropriate circumstances. Indeed, she had two road traffic accidents and stopped driving. Witnesses report that she 'looks asleep', and that there is no period of absence and no convulsive features. On direct questioning, she denies falls triggered by emotional factors, sleep paralysis or vivid dreams. She has no other medical history and there is no family history of similar problems. She takes no regular medication.

Systemic and neurological examination is entirely normal. Metabolic screening (urea and electrolytes, renal, thyroid and liver function and full blood count) were normal. Waking EEG revealed excessive levels of drowsiness but was otherwise normal.

(a) Name two causes of this presentation.
(b) How should she be investigated?

Answer 23

(a) Idiopathic hypersomnia.
   Narcoleptic syndrome.
(b) Sleep EEG.
   Human leucocyte antigen (HLA) typing.

Comment

Metabolic causes of hypersomnolence have been excluded and there are no clinical features to support a diagnosis of epilepsy. In patients with the narcoleptic syndrome, the gap between the onset of excessive daytime sleepiness and cataplexy is usually less than 2 years but may be much longer. Accordingly, both symptoms are usually reported at initial presentation. However, in the absence of cataplexy, confident clinical diagnosis is difficult.

Excessive daytime somnolence occurs in 0.3–4% of the population. Most cases are not due to the narcoleptic syndrome, but the existence of 'monosymptomatic narcolepsy' – excessive daytime somnolence plus sleep-onset rapid eye movement (REM) sleep – is generally accepted. This should be differentiated from idiopathic hypersomnia in the young, and obstructive sleep apnoea in the middle aged/elderly, especially males. The distinction depends on clinical features, particularly identification of the pathological nature of the sleepiness, sleep laboratory findings and HLA typing. Sleep paralysis occurs in two-thirds of those with narcoleptic syndrome, 5–10% obstructive sleep apnoea but rarely in idiopathic hypersomnia. While the resting EEG is normal, overnight recordings reveal short sleep latency, frequent awakenings and fragmented REM sleep. The absence of HLA DR2 on tissue typing, present in > 90% of those with the narcoleptic syndrome, mitigates against this diagnosis.

Question 24

A 70 year old man with severe ischaemic heart disease became aware of increasing tiredness, coldness of his extremities, pallor and loss of body hair. Attributing these symptoms to his age and general ill-health, he did not report them to his general practitioner.

He was admitted for coronary artery bypass grafting which was apparently uncomplicated. Postoperatively he spent 24 hours in an intensive care unit before being transferred to a ward where he reported right periorbital pain.

Examination revealed a right-sided ptosis and complete ophthalmoplegia. However, after a CT scan was reported to be normal, he was returned to his local hospital. Subsequent neurological examination confirmed the original findings, noted that the pupil was mid-sized and fixed, and, in addition, noted impaired sensation on the right side of his forehead and a left temporal visual field defect. Incidentally, general examination revealed that he was pale with smooth skin and there was a distinct lack of facial hair.

(a) Where is the lesion?
(b) What is the mechanism of his sudden deterioration?

Answer 24

(a) Pituitary lesion invading the right cavernous sinus.
(b) Intraoperative infarction and swelling of this lesion.

Comment

The presence of a unilateral ptosis, total ophthalmoplegia and impaired sensation in the distribution of the ophthalmic division of the trigeminal nerve represents a complete cavernous sinus syndrome. The fixed, mid-sized pupil is a consequence of paralysis of both the sympathetic and parasympathetic nerve supply to the pupil. The additional finding of a left temporal field defect and clinical features of hypopituitarism indicate a lesion arising from the pituitary fossa invading the cavernous sinus. At operation, there was clear evidence of a haemorrhagic infarct within the tumour which is likely to have been the consequence of profound hypotension during the coronary artery bypass graft.

Question 25

A 57 year old heavy goods vehicle driver developed an aching sensation around his right elbow radiating to the right wrist and fingers. Over the next few weeks he developed worsening numbness of both hands, the left foot and then the right foot. His gait became increasingly unsteady and he had several falls.

He had no medical history of note nor occupational exposure to neurotoxic chemicals. He smoked heavily (30 cigarettes per day) but, apart from a smoker's cough, he had no chest symptoms and was systemically well.

He appeared generally well. Examination of the chest, cardiovascular system and abdomen was entirely normal. His gait was ataxic but there was no muscle weakness. Upper limb reflexes were present but lower limb reflexes were absent. There was marked impairment of joint position sense at the hallux bilaterally, diminished cutaneous perception to pin prick and light touch distal to the wrists, the left foot and most of the right leg.

Nerve conduction studies revealed a sensory axonopathy with normal motor conduction. The following tests were normal or negative: FBC, ESR, urea electrolytes, fasting sugar, liver function tests, serum B12 and red cell folate, serum immunoglobulins and protein electrophoresis, antinuclear factor, autoantibodies and tests for extractable nuclear antigens. CSF protein was elevated at 0.7 g/l, but there were no cells and cytocentrifuge revealed no malignant cells.

(a) What is the likeliest diagnosis?
(b) Which immunological test might support this diagnosis?
(c) Which non-neurological investigation is essential?

Answer 25

(a) Paraneoplastic neuropathy.
(b) Anti-hu antibody.
(c) Chest X-ray or CT scan of chest.

Comment

The clinical picture of a subacute purely sensory axonopathy (dorsal root ganglionitis) is highly suggestive of a paraneoplastic phenomenon which most commonly occurs in association with an occult oat cell carcinoma of the lung.

Antineuronal antibodies (anti-hu), when present in high titre, support the diagnosis even if the chest X-ray or CT scan of the chest are normal at presentation.

The neuropathy may proceed the clinical manifestations of the primary tumour by months or even years and, indeed, the neuropathy may improve if the primary lesion can be resected. Otherwise, although spontaneous remissions can occur and there are anecdotal reports of temporary improvements with intravenous immunoglobulin, in most cases the neurological disability is relentlessly progressive.

Question 26

A 60 year old woman presented with bradykinesia, postural instability and falls. Her motor disability was progressive from onset and poorly responsive to Sinemet Plus one tablet tds. Her husband had noted apathy, lack of spontaneous speech and, at times, disorientation.

There was no antecedent history of psychiatric illness or exposure to psychotropic medication, no history of stroke, head trauma or vascular risk factors.

Her blood pressure fluctuated from 160–180/80–110 but there was no consistent evidence of postural hypotension. Mini mental score was 20/30. She had expressionless facies with a fixed stare and she was slow to respond to command. There was an impairment of up and down gaze, and dysarthria of the extrapyramidal type. She had no involuntary movements, but she had symmetrical rigidity of all four limbs and prominent axial rigidity. There was a mild degree of spasticity with brisk reflexes and flexor plantar responses. Her gait was shuffling with a tendency to fall backwards.

FBC, ESR, biochemistry and serological tests for syphilis were normal. Her MRI scan revealed a moderate degree of generalized atrophy but no focal abnormalities.

What is the diagnosis?

Answer 26

Steel–Richardson–Oslewski syndrome (progressive supranuclear palsy).

Comment

The presentation with falls, symmetrical extrapyramidal signs and poor response to levodopa militates strongly against the diagnosis of idiopathic Parkinson's disease. The prominent axial rigidity, early development of cognitive decline, of subcortical type, and impairment of vertical gaze point to the diagnosis of progressive supranuclear palsy. It is important to recognize that impairment of up gaze is an age-related phenomenon whilst impairment of down gaze is a characteristic feature of this condition.

The absence of focal lesions on the MRI scan excludes the alternative possibility of diffuse subcortical ischaemia which can mimic this condition.

There may be an incomplete symptomatic response to higher doses of levodopa (Sinemet 275 tds) but the overall prognosis is poor with increasing disability culminating in death usually within 5 years.

Question 27

Whilst on holiday, a 59 year old man walked into someone whom he had not seen. He did not check his vision at that time. However, on his return, he found vision in his right eye to be 'hazy'.

In the previous year, he had two episodes of 'loss of vision' in the left eye. He was seen in the ophthalmology clinic and advised to stop smoking and started on aspirin.

His blood pressure was 150/90, with a regular pulse and normal heart sounds. He had a right homonymous inferior quadrantanopia but there were no other neurological signs.

FBC, ESR and fasting glucose were normal, but random cholesterol was elevated.

(a) Where is the intracranial lesion?
(b) What extracranial lesion should be excluded?

Question 28

A 48 year old foreman had a blackout whilst walking home from the pub. He could recall no warning and his first clear memory was of being in the ambulance. There were no definite convulsive features.

The casualty notes included the comments 'smells strongly of alcohol', 'CVS – NAD' and 'CNS – no focal signs'. He was referred to the neurology clinic with a diagnosis of a first fit.

He admitted to shortness of breath on exertion but attributed this to smoking 30–40 cigarettes per day. He also admitted to drinking 5–6 pints of beer per day.

Examination revealed a blood pressure of 110/80, a low volume radial pulse, and a systolic murmur heard all over the precordium and radiating to the neck. Neurological examination was entirely normal.

What is the diagnosis?

Answer 27

(a) Left parietal lobe.
(b) > 70% left internal carotid artery stenosis.

Comment

The upper fibres of the optic radiation, carrying visual information from the contralateral lower quadrant, are situated in the parietal lobe. This part of the brain may take its vascular supply from either the anterior (carotid) or posterior (vertebro-basilar) circulation. Given the history suggestive of left amaurosis fugax and the occurrence of a left hemisphere stroke, despite taking aspirin, a significant (> 70%) internal carotid artery stenosis should be excluded. Carotid endarterectomy reduces the risk of ischaemic stroke by 75% in the first 2–3 years after surgery. In expert hands, the operation itself carries less than 3% risk of perioperative stroke.

Answer 28

Severe aortic stenosis.

Comment

Always keep an open mind. Any adult presenting with blackouts without convincing features of a convulsive seizure should be questioned about cardiac symptoms and examined for signs. In the vast majority of cases, there will be historical or circumstantial features pointing to a diagnosis of simple syncope and examination will be normal. If these features are absent, cardiology assessment is essential. Occasionally, as in this case, there will be clear-cut evidence of cardiac pathology. The combination of left ventricular outflow obstruction and the vasodilatory effect of alcohol caused a critical fall in the cardiac output, leading to abrupt loss of consciousness.

Cardiac catheterization confirmed the presence of critical aortic stenosis, with a gradient of 120 mmHg, necessitating aortic valve replacement.

Question 29

A 51 year old ambulance man was admitted to an orthopaedic ward with a 3-week history of low back pain, an aching sensation in the anterior aspect of the right thigh and heaviness of both feet. Prior to admission he developed numbness in a median nerve distribution bilaterally. Whilst in hospital, his lower limb weakness progressed to the extent that he was unable to stand.

Past medical history included late-onset, drug-resistant asthma requiring chronic steroid therapy. He had been investigated for proteinuria and found to have only one kidney.

On transfer to a neurological unit, he was found to have a blood pressure of 120/80, a tachycardia of 130 and soft normal heart sounds. His chest was hyperinflated but clear, and his abdomen was normal. Cranial nerves were also normal. He had mild weakness of intrinsic hand muscles bilaterally and a severe bilateral foot drop. Upper limb and left knee jerks were present, while right knee jerk and both ankle jerks were absent.

There was impaired cutaneous perception to pin prick in the distribution of both median nerves, the right medial cutaneous nerve of thigh and the right common peroneal nerve.

Electrophysiology confirmed the clinical suspicion of mononeuritis multiplex. Haemoglobin and platelet counts were normal, but white blood count was elevated with an eosinophilia varying from 15% to 19%. Urea and electrolytes were normal but urinary protein level was elevated and serum albumin reduced. Antinuclear factor, autoantibodies, antineutrophil cytoplasmic antibody (ANCA) and tests for extractable nuclear antigens were all negative. Chest X-ray revealed cardiomegaly, which, on echocardiogram, proved to be a localized effusion not amenable to pericardiocentesis.

He was treated aggressively and, after transfer to his local hospital, he could walk with elbow crutches.

(a) What was the aggressive treatment?
(b) What is the prognosis?

Answer 29

(a) Steroids plus cyclophosphamide.
(b) Poor – 50% mortality within 5 years.

Comment

The clinical picture of late-onset, drug-resistant asthma, eosinophilia, proteinuria, cardiac and neurological problems is highly suggestive of polyarteritis nodosa. Mononeuritis multiplex is the commonest neurological manifestation of this condition. Biopsy of a sural nerve, revealing a perineural inflammatory infiltrate consisting of mononuclear cells and eosinophils, was consistent with this diagnosis. Many vasculitic neuropathies do not respond to steroids but do respond to cyclophosphamide. Nevertheless, the prognosis for survival is poor with a mortality of 50% within 5 years.

Question 30

For approximately 4 years, a middle-aged man had been aware of a tendency to trip. During the previous 12 months, he had developed a gradually progressive right-sided neurological deficit comprising dragging and clumsiness of his leg, 'numbness' of the leg, trunk and hand, and weakness of grip.

He was generally well with no medical or family history of note.

Systematic examination and cranial nerves were normal. He had a mild right hemiparesis with weakness of shoulder abduction and absence of right arm reflexes. There was patchy diminution of perception of light touch over the right leg, trunk and arm, impairment of pin prick and temperature sensation to a level just above the left nipple and diminished joint position sense at the right ankle and, to a lesser extent, the right thumb.

Where is the lesion?

Question 31

One morning, after washing the dishes and doing some ironing, a 49 year old woman became giddy and so unsteady that she fell several times on the way to work. She had also experienced the curious notion that someone familiar was standing beside her but nothing was visible. She was sent home because of weakness of her left arm and face. After 'sleeping it off', she awoke feeling disorientated and was admitted to hospital.

On admission she was alert and orientated with no signs other than unsteadiness on her feet. Cardiovascular examination was normal.

Full blood count, biochemistry, including sugar and cholesterol, and CT scan of the brain were normal. Because of 'visual hallucinations' she was referred to a psychiatrist who found her mental state to be entirely normal. She was given a diagnosis of TIA, advised to stop smoking and discharged on aspirin. Subsequent investigation included a negative thrombophilia screen and echocardiogram, but MRI scan revealed a few high-intensity lesions in the cerebral hemispheres suggestive of ischaemia.

She was reviewed again by a neurologist. Neurological examination was normal. Blood pressure was 150/80 mmHg in the right arm and heart sounds were normal. Further examination revealed signs which could explain the initial presentation.

(a) Which other clinical signs were elicited?
(b) Give a possible mechanism for her 'stroke'.

Answer 30

Right mid-cervical cord (C 5 level).

Comment

This man has a partial/incomplete right Brown–Sequard syndrome. This comprises ipsilateral pyramidal and dorsal column signs with contralateral spinothalamic sensory loss. Weakness of shoulder abduction and absence of biceps jerk localizes the lesion to the right mid-cervical region at the C5 level.

The complete syndrome is relatively rare, since structural lesions often affect parts of both sides of the cord. Therefore, partial syndromes often produce bilateral, asymmetric motor and sensory signs. Because light touch is supplied by fibres of both spinothalamic and dorsal columns, loss of this sensory modality implies that this lesion is compressing both sides of the cord.

The mode of onset implies progressive intrinsic cord pathology. Ependymomas and astrocytomas are the commonest intramedullary tumours, but this patient had a haemangioblastoma which was completely excised.

Answer 31

(a) Low volume left radial pulse, low blood pressure in the left arm and left subclavian bruit.
(b) Subclavian steal.

Comment

The history of vertigo, ataxia and left-sided weakness suggest ischaemia in the vertebrobasilar territory. Transient memory impairment, owing to reduced flow in the posterior cerebral artery, which supplies the hippocampus, is an uncommon but well-recognized feature.

Examination revealed signs of a left subclavian artery stenosis: weak left radial pulse, blood pressure equal to 70/40 mmHg in the left arm and a subclavian bruit. When the subclavian artery is blocked proximal to the origin of the vertebral artery, exercise of the ipsilateral arm draws blood from the vertebrobasilar system into the arm, producing symptoms of basilar insufficiency. Medical treatment is recommended but, if TIAs occur despite aspirin, subclavian angioplasty should be considered.

Question 32

A 22 year old man presented with a short history of headaches, vomiting and ataxia. He had no significant medical history but his father died, in his thirties, from a cerebral haemorrhage. The patient was married with two children aged 7 and 5.

Examination revealed papilloedema and left-sided cerebellar signs. The remainder of the routine neurological and systematic examination was normal.

An MRI scan showed a left cerebellar tumour which was resected and proved to be a haemangioblastoma. He made a complete recovery.

What are the implications of this presentation for:

(a) The patient;
(b) His children?

Answer 32

(a) He has a 20% chance of having Von Hippel–Lindau disease.
(b) If the patient has this disease, his children have a 50% chance of inheriting the condition.

Comment

Von Hippel–Landau (VHL) disease, defined as two or more haemangioblastomas, is an autosomal dominant condition with variable expression. Multiple lesions occur in 60% of cases and retinal lesions in 50%. There is a significant risk of renal carcinoma which increases with age and other associations include phaeochromocytoma, hepatic, renal and pancreatic cysts, and epididymal tumours.

Cerebellar haemangioblastomas account for 10% of all posterior fossa tumours. Most present in the fourth decade but earlier in patients with VHL disease. Any index case, with a negative family history, should be vigorously screened. Unfortunately, there are no skin markers and, while the condition has been linked to chromosome 3, there is no specific diagnostic test.

Screening should include an ophthalmology assessment with fluorescein retinal angiography, abdominal CT scan, vanillyl mandelic acids (VMAs) and epididymal ultrasound. If screening is negative, the patient should be followed up indefinitely and rescreened on suspicion. If the index case has VHL disease, he or she should be screened at intervals and his or her children should also be screened. This is particularly important because the commonest presentation in childhood is blindness, which can be prevented by photocoagulation of retinal lesions.

Question 33

A 55 year old dairy farmer presented with a 6-month history of progressive difficulty walking. His legs ached particularly after exertion. He had no back pain or sphincter disturbance. He had no previous neurological symptoms and no family history of neurological disease. He denied exposure to neurotoxic chemicals.

General examination was entirely normal. He had mild spasticity of his legs with preservation of power and no sensory signs.

The following investigations were normal/negative: spinal cord and brain MRI, whole spine myelogram, CSF examination, visual evoked responses, EMG and nerve conduction studies (NCS), blood count, ESR, renal and liver function, serum B_{12} and red cell folate, antinuclear factor and autoantibodies, tests for extractable nuclear antigens and serological tests for syphilis. He was discharged without a specific diagnosis.

Three months later he had deteriorated. Repeat examination revealed no wasting or fasiculation. Cranial nerves and upper limbs were normal. Lower limb spasticity had increased and he had mild weakness in a pyramidal distribution.

Repeat MRI of spinal cord and EMG/NCS were negative as were serological tests for borrelia, human immunodeficiency virus (HIV) and human T-cell leukaemia virus-1 (HTLV1), very long chain fatty acid levels and tests for antineuronal antibodies. An ophthalmology assessment was satisfactory and a labial gland biopsy was normal.

(a) Into which 'broad' diagnostic category should he be placed?
(b) Suggest three 'specific' diagnostic possibilities.

Answer 33

(a) Myelopathy of unknown cause.
(b) Motor neurone disease, hereditary spastic paraparesis, primary lateral sclerosis.

Comment

Spastic paraparesis is a common presentation. Compressive, vascular, demyelinating, infective, deficiency states and toxic causes have been excluded. A paraneoplastic process was considered but seems unlikely. Adrenoleucodystrophy very rarely presents in midlife but is effectively excluded by the normal MRI and very long chain fatty acid levels.

This situation is regularly encountered in neurological practice. In some cases, lower motor neurone signs develop and subsequent EMGs reveal evidence of anterior horn cell disease. Two diagnoses of exclusion should be considered. Hereditary spastic paraparesis is a dominantly inherited condition characterized by extreme spasticity and relative preservation of power. However, sporadic cases occur and late onset may be associated with a more aggressive clinical course. Primary lateral sclerosis is a purely upper motor neurone disorder with normal EMG and imaging. Recent evidence suggests that MRI, in the coronal plane, through the motor gyrus, may reveal atrophic changes. The condition is slowly progressive and probably accounts for some 'long survivors with motor neurone disease'. Despite the passage of time, the cause of spastic paraparesis cannot be established in 10–15% of cases.

Question 34

A 61 year old man developed acute myeloid leukaemia. He entered remission after three pulses of MAC (mitrozantone and cytosine arabinoside). Subsequently, he received three pulses of CHOP (cyclophosphamide, vincristine, cytosine arabinoside and prednisolone) and, after haematological parameters returned to normal, regular subcutaneous interferon.

During treatment, he developed lumbar discomfort radiating to the groin and subsequently sensory symptoms and weakness affecting, in order, the left arm, right arm and both legs.

Examination of the cranial nerves was normal. He had a flaccid, areflexic tetraparesis with patchy reduction of light touch, pin prick and temperature of all four limbs, but preservation of vibration and joint position sense.

Investigation revealed the following results: white cell count $2.9 \times 10^9/l$, haemoglobin 13.5 g/l, platelets $156 \times 10^9/l$. Bone marrow biopsy confirmed that the leukaemia was in remission. CSF protein was slightly elevated at 0.56 g/l but there were no cells.

(a) What is the likeliest diagnosis?
(b) What treatment is required?

Answer 34

(a) Leukaemic infiltration of spinal nerve roots.
(b) Radiotherapy to the whole neuraxis and intrathecal chemotherapy.

Comment

When a patient suffering from leukaemia develops neurological symptoms, the differential diagnosis rests between leukaemic infiltration of the nervous system and neurotoxicity due to the chemotherapeutic agents. This distinction is important because neurotoxicity necessitates cessation of the offending drug while infiltration demands aggressive local treatment. It is important to recognize that neurological relapse can occur in the presence of haemotological remission and that, if leukaemic infiltration involves the proximal parts of cranial nerves or spinal roots, there may be no blast cells on CSF examination.

In this case, EMG revealed widespread denervation of limb and paraspinal muscles with virtually normal peripheral motor and sensory nerve conduction. An alternative method of establishing the diagnosis is MRI, with and without gadolinium, which will usually reveal enhancement of affected nerve roots. Treatment involves radiotherapy to the whole neuraxis and intrathecal chemotherapy.

Question 35

A 26 year old pharmacist was referred for a second neurological opinion. After being admitted with chest pain, she had had an episode of collapse. Thereafter, she continued to experience blackouts, some of which were preceded by 'butterflies in the stomach' and a visual disturbance. She was always observed to shake but there was no tongue biting or cyanosis. After the shaking subsided, she could be unresponsive for up to an hour. Her attacks did not respond to antiepileptic drugs. They tended to occur in series, often resulting in hospitalization and usually occurring in association with other physical symptoms.

Her past medical history was complex. She had irritable bowel syndrome (abdominal pain, nausea, altered bowel habit), recurrent urinary tract infection (UTI; frequency, dysuria) and episodes of urinary retention requiring self-catheterization, chest pains and shortness of breath diagnosed as pulmonary emboli, and joint pains diagnosed as systemic lupus erythematosus (SLE). There was no history of cerebral insult. She had taken one overdose but had no other psychiatric history.

Systemic and neurological examination was normal. Previous cerebral imaging had been normal and, during ambulatory monitoring, there was no electrical correlate of her usual attacks.

She was admitted for video telemetry but had no attacks. Review of her records from three other hospitals revealed that autoimmune screening had been negative on three occasions, V/Q scans had been normal on six occasions and thorough investigation of her urinary tract had revealed no structural or neurological abnormality.

What is the likeliest diagnosis?

Answer 35

Somatization disorder.

Comment

The nervous system lends itself to non-organic presentations of which pseu-doseizures represent a common example. Factors supporting the diagnosis in this case include female sex, paramedical occupation, late onset without apparent cause, variability of attacks and lack of response to antiepileptic drugs.

In cases where pseudoseizures represent a response to a recent emotional trauma, the prognosis is excellent. In those with a history of a traumatic childhood, psychiatric problems, especially deliberate self-harm, and unex-plained physical symptoms, there is likely to be significant underlying psychopathology associated with a much poorer outcome. A proportion of these patients satisfy the DSM-IV* criteria for somatization disorder: at least 2 years of multiple and variable unexplained physical symptoms, preoccupation with symptoms causing distress and stimulating repeated medical consultations, and persistent reluctance to accept that symptoms do not have a physical basis. If these patients can be persuaded to accept a psychological basis for the physical symptoms, cognitive behavioural therapy may help.

*Diagnostic and Statistic Manual IV. This is the American classification of psychiatric conditions which is accepted internationally for purposes of research.

Question 36

A 62 year old woman reported a gradually progressive reduction of mobility. Specifically she complained of tiredness and aching in the calves, which limited her walking distance to 200 metres, but which was relieved by rest. Occasionally, she had sharp pain which radiated down the posterior aspect of her thighs and lateral aspect of her lower legs. She had a long history of intermittent neck and low back pain.

Despite requiring nifedipine for hypertension and isosorbide mononitrate for angina, she had continued to smoke 20 cigarettes daily.

Tone was minimally increased in all four limbs. There was isolated weakness of the left extensor hallucis longus. Upper limb and knee jerks were symmetrically brisk, ankle jerks were absent but plantar responses were unequivocally extensor. Dorsalis pedis pulses were palpable.

(a) How is this combination of clinical signs explained?
(b) Where is the symptomatic lesion?

Question 37

For several years a 55 year old man had experienced brief episodes of intense vertigo and nausea triggered by head movement and, particularly, when lying on his left side. He denied dysarthria, diplopia or lateralized limb symptoms. Attacks had increased in frequency despite trials of stemetil and serc. Between attacks he was perfectly well and his hearing was entirely normal.

Neurological examination and audiometry were normal.

Positional testing was performed: in the left head-hanging position with gaze to the left, after an interval of 20 seconds, symptoms occurred and torsional nystagmus was observed. With gaze to the right vertical nystagmus was noted. On repeat testing, no nystagmus was seen.

What is the most likely diagnosis?

Answer 36

(a) Cervical myelopathy and lumbar canal stenosis.
(b) Lumbar canal stenosis at L5/S1 level.

Comment

Cervical spondylosis with cord compression and lumbar spondylosis with nerve root compression is the commonest cause of absent ankle jerks and extensor plantar responses. The myelopathy, while responsible for the brisk reflexes and extensor plantar responses, is asymptomatic. The patient is describing claudication, which, in the presence of palpable pedal pulses, is neurogenic. Weakness of extensor hallucis longus (L5) and absent ankle jerks localize the canal stenosis to the L5/S1 level. Lumbar canal decompression is usually highly effective.

Answer 37

Benign paroxysmal positional vertigo.

Comment

Patients with vertigo are commonly referred to neurologists for exclusion of central causes. However, central positional vertigo is uncommon. In patients with chronic posterior fossa lesions, other symptoms usually predominate. On positional testing, nystagmus is unidirectional, occurs immediately, persists and does not attenuate on repeat testing. Isolated vertigo rarely occurs as the sole manifestation of vertebrobasilar ischaemia but progression to brainstem stroke usually occurs within a few months (rarely as long as 2 years).

Benign positional paroxysmal vertigo is probably the commonest cause of vertigo in middle age. Unlike Ménière's disease, hearing is unaffected. Positional testing reveals nystagmus, with latency to onset, tendency to fatigue and attenuation on repeat testing. The condition usually occurs spontaneously but can be the consequence of viral labyrinthitis, trauma or ischaemic lesions of the labyrinth. Attacks do not respond to vestibular sedatives. Recent evidence suggests that the mechanism is displacement of otoconia from the utricle of the macula in the semicircular canals, usually the posterior canal. These otoconia have been seen at surgery and symptoms have been relieved after their removal. However, in expert hands, physical therapy (canalith repositioning manoeuvres) can abolish symptoms in 50–80% of cases.

Question 38

A 26 year old homosexual, known to be HIV positive, with a history of *Pneumocystis carinii* pneumonia, was admitted to hospital with a 2–3 week history of progressive right-sided weakness. He complained of mild generalized headache, fever and chills.

Examination revealed that he was marginally febrile ($T = 37.8°C$) with no skin lesions, mild generalized adenopathy but no organomegaly.

Investigation revealed mild pancytopenia with a CD4 count (number of T-helper cells) of 350. CT and MRI showed a contrast-enhancing lesion, with mass effect, in the left hemisphere. Toxoplasma serology was positive.

(a) Which two conditions should be considered?
(b) Name three non-invasive methods of distinguishing between the two possibilities.

Question 39

An elderly man, with a long history of idiopathic Parkinson's disease, remained independently mobile but reported a 6-month history of progressive difficulty using his hands which had not improved since pergolide was added to his dopamine replacement therapy. Specifically, he had difficulty telling that objects were in his hands and had to look at them in order to use them. Consequently, he had problems using a fork and knife, tying shoe laces, etc. On direct questioning, he admitted to neck pain but no radicular pain.

Examination revealed cog-wheel rigidity at the wrist but no spasticity, and power was normal in all muscle groups. Upper limb reflexes were brisk with a right-sided Hoffman's jerk, while lower limb reflexes were normal and plantar responses flexor. While light touch and joint position sense in the hands appeared normal, he had difficulty fastening buttons with his eyes closed.

Which treatable condition should be excluded?

Answer 38

(a) Toxoplasma abscess and cerebral lymphoma.
(b) Epstein–Barr virus (EBV) serology, thallium scan and response to anti-toxoplasma therapy.

Comment

In this context, toxoplasma abscess and cerebral lymphoma are clinically indistinguishable and cerebral imaging can be very similar. CD4 count tends to be lower in patients with a lymphoma but this feature does not differentiate between the two conditions. While toxoplasma serology could be coincidental, EBV serology is strongly associated with lymphoma. Furthermore, lymphomas appear 'hot' on thallium scanning. In practical terms, the response to a 2-week trial of antitoxoplasma therapy is recommended. If no response occurs, biopsy will distinguish between non-responding toxoplasmosis and lymphoma. In the latter case and, if the patient is in good condition, steroids and radiotherapy will alleviate the focal deficit but the long-term prognosis is poor.

Answer 39

High cervical myelopathy.

Comment

The striking feature in this case is the inconsistency between his mobility and the problems with his hands, suggesting that these symptoms are unrelated to the Parkinson's disease. He is, in fact, describing 'numb clumsy hands', a presentation highly suggestive of a high cervical myelopathy. The other clinical findings are highly variable; there may be few signs of cord compression and, therefore, investigations should be based on the symptoms alone. His MRI confirmed spondylitic cord compression at C3/4 which was successfully decompressed with improvement in hand function. Why lesions at this level can produce proprioceptive deficits with relative sparing of motor function is not well understood.

Question 40

A 52 year old alcoholic woman was admitted to hospital with a minor head injury. She suffered from epilepsy which was well controlled with phenytoin 300 mg nocte.

On examination, she was clearly intoxicated but well orientated with no focal deficits. A skull X-ray revealed no fracture.

During the next 48 hours she became more confused. She was unsteady with horizontal nystagmus bilaterally but no focal signs. No seizures had been witnessed. Her EEG revealed no epileptiform discharges and there was no focal pathology on CT. Metabolic screen was normal and phenytoin levels were within the target range.

(a) What is the diagnosis?
(b) What treatment is indicated?

Answer 40

(a) Wernicke's encephalopathy.
(b) High-dose intravenous thiamine.

Comment

In the head-injured alcoholic, persisting confusion should never be attributed to the residual effects of the head injury and intoxication. In this case, the normal CT and EEG excluded subdural haematoma and non-convulsive status epilepticus, respectively.

While the possibility of phenytoin toxicity was entertained, Wernicke's encephalopathy is the likeliest explanation. The full picture comprises ataxia, gaze palsies and confusion, but these can occur singly or in any combination. Therefore, this condition should be suspected in any confused alcoholic and intravenous thiamine administered immediately. The prognosis is poor, especially if treatment is delayed. The mortality rate in the acute phase is 10–20%. Most (80%) survivors develop features of Korsakoff's psychosis (anterograde and retrograde amnesia with or without confabulation), while up to 60% retain features of acute Wernicke's encephalopathy, particularly ataxia and nystagmus. Consequently, many of these individuals become dependent on institutionalized care.

Data Interpretation

Question 1

A 43 year old man presented with a 9-year history of blackouts preceded by a sensation of light-headedness. Witnesses reported a brief period of staring and profound pallor while he was unconscious. The attacks did not respond to a 'therapeutic trial' of carbamazepine. During an ambulatory EEG, a typical symptomatic event was captured.

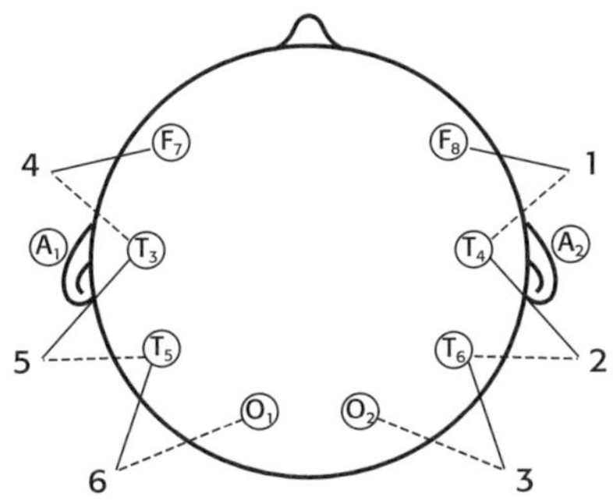

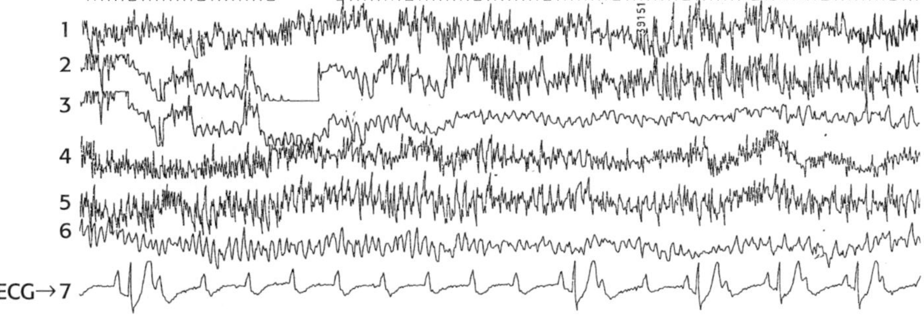

(a) What is the cause of his blackouts?
(b) Name two aspects of management.

Question 2

This is the EEG of a 10 year old boy who has 'not been paying attention' in his classes at school.

The EEG montage is transverse with four across the front (2R, 2L), six across the middle (3R, 3L) and six across the back (3R, 3L) of the head.

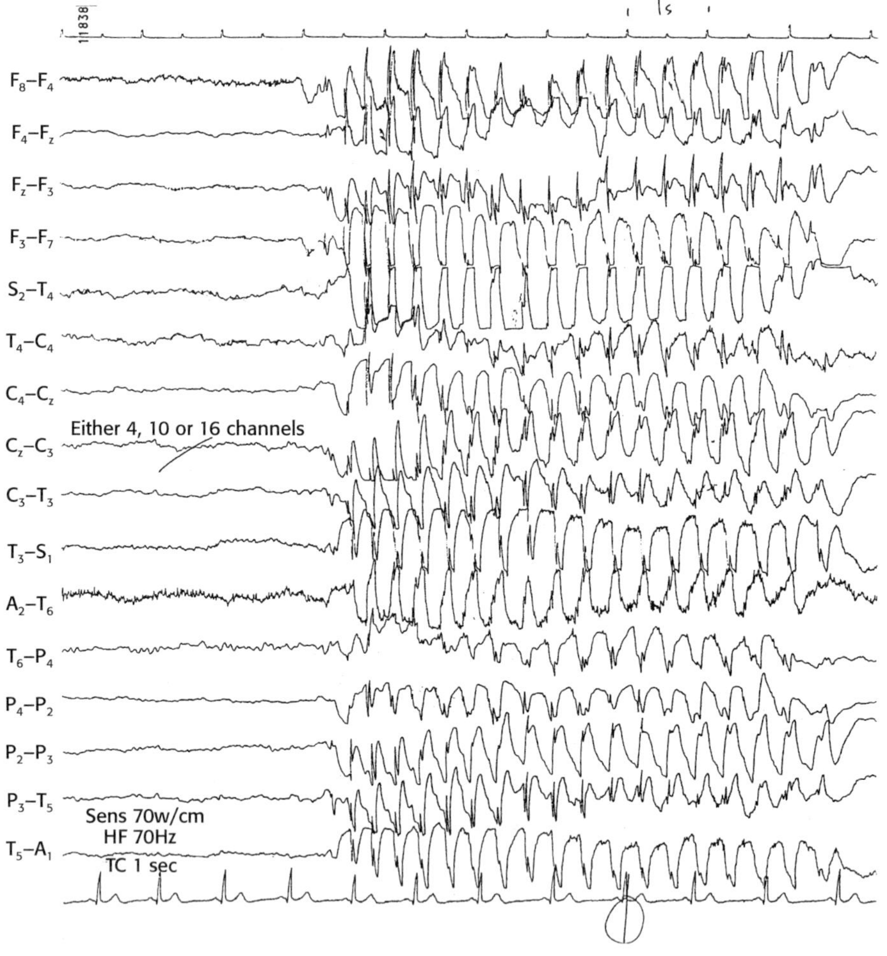

(a) What is this abnormality?
(b) Which drug is only effective against the seizures associated with this EEG abnormality?

Question 3

A 72 year old man developed profound limb weakness and oliguria 1 week after a flu-like illness. Examination revealed proximal weakness which was more marked in the lower limbs. Knee reflexes were absent but all other reflexes were present, plantar responses were flexor and there were no sensory signs.

His biochemical profile was as follows:

Urea	54 mmol/l
Creatinine	783 μmol/l
Potassium	7.9 mmol/l
Sodium	132 mmol/l
Total bilirubin	17 μmol/l
AST	2100 IU/l
ALT	1200 IU/l
GGT	46 IU/l
Alkaline phosphatase	115 IU/l
CPK	87 000 IU/l

How may the clinical and biochemical presentation be explained?

Question 4

A 28 year old intravenous drug abuser was admitted to hospital with a 3-week history of headache. He was febrile ($T = 38.0°C$) with mild neck stiffness but no other neurological signs, and CT scan of brain was normal. Systematic examination was normal but he was found to be HIV positive.

CSF examination produced the following results:

Protein	0.58 g/l
Red cell count	$< 5/mm^3$
White cell count	$32/mm^3$
	(80% lymphocytes)
Glucose	3.5 mmol/l
	(Blood glucose 6.2 mmol/l)
Gram stain	Negative
Ziehl–Nielsen stain	Negative
TPHA, VDRL	Negative

Which infective cause should be actively sought?

Question 5

A 75 year old man presented with a 6-month history of progressive weakness and numbness affecting all four limbs. Examination revealed signs of a predominantly motor neuropathy, worse in the legs, which was confirmed by nerve conduction studies. Haematological, biochemical and immunological screening was normal.

The results of CSF examination were:

Protein	1.2 g/l
White cells	$< 5/mm^3$
Red cells	$< 5/mm^3$
Glucose	3.4 mmol/l
	(Blood glucose 6.2 mmol/l)

(a) What is the most likely diagnosis?
(b) What is the treatment of first choice?

Question 6

A middle-aged woman presented with progressive painless proximal limb weakness which was confirmed on examination. The rest of systematic examination including skin and joints was normal. Full blood count, urea and creatinine, sodium, potassium, calcium, phosphate, glucose and thyroid function were normal. She denied alcohol excess but because of deranged 'liver function tests' (shown below), she underwent a liver biopsy which was also normal.

INR	1.1
APTT	1.2
Albumin	40 g/l
Bilirubin	23 mmol/l
AST	356 IU/l
ALT	217 IU/l
Alkaline phosphatase	204 IU/l

(a) What is the diagnosis?
(b) Which two simple blood tests would have been more useful than a liver biopsy?
(c) What is the treatment?

Question 7

This is part of an EEG recording performed on a psychiatric in-patient with a 3-month history of increasing confusion. Examination revealed that she was disorientated in time, place and person, and that she appeared to be blind but retinae, optic discs and pupillary reactions were all normal.

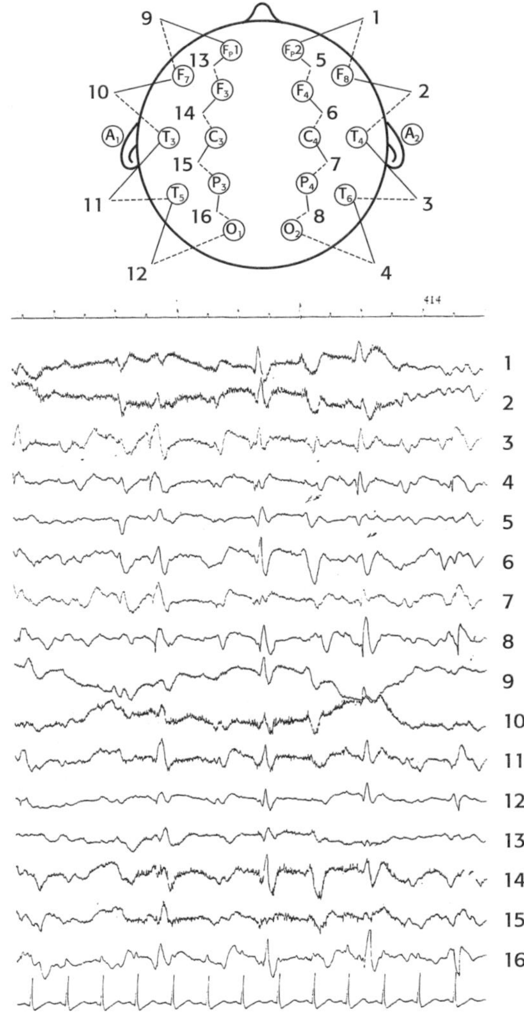

(a) What is the abnormality?
(b) What diagnosis should be considered?

Question 8

A 48 year old woman was admitted to a neurological ward because of progressive generalized weakness. She reported a short history of palpitations, shortness of breath, weight loss and insomnia. Examination revealed a fine tremor, bounding tachycardia, a mild degree of heart failure and proximal limb weakness, and EMG revealed myopathic changes. Her biochemical profile was unremarkable (see below).

Urea	10.1 mmol/l
Creatinine	141 μmol/l
Sodium	144 mmol/l
Potassium	4.4 mmol/l
Calcium	2.24 mmol/l
Phosphate	1.38 mmol/l
Bilirubin	31 μmol/l
AST	58 IU/l
ALT	46 IU/l
Alkaline phosphate	110 IU/l
Total protein	78 g/l
Albumin	35 g/l
CPK	160 IU/l
Free T4	19 pmol/l
TSH	1.8 mU/l

Which other blood test should have been requested?

Question 9

These are the relevant visual evoked responses (VERs) of a 29 year old woman, with no previous neurological problems, who presented with a subacute spastic paraparesis and whose MRI scan of the spine was normal.

	Major positive first peak latency (ms)
Right eye	122
Left eye	98
Normal range	95–110

What is the implication of this result?

Question 10

During the course of a mild upper respiratory tract infection, an 8 year old boy was admitted to hospital with profuse vomiting, fever and confusion. Investigations revealed the following results:

Venous blood

Urea	11.2 mmol/l
Creatinine	143 μmol/l
Sodium	146 mmol/l
Potassium	4.7 mmol/l
Glucose	2.3 mmol/l
Bilirubin	31 μmol/l
AST	624 IU/l
ALT	730 IU/l

Arterial blood

pH	7.27
pCO_2	42 mmHg
pO_2	96 mmHg
Base excess	−1.2 mmol/l
Std bicarbonate	17 mmol/l

CSF

Protein	52 mg/dl
White cells	$< 5/mm^3$
Glucose	1.2 mmol/l (blood glucose 2.7 mmol/l)

(a) What is the diagnosis?
(b) Which other blood test is indicated?

Question 11

A 36 year old male homosexual was transferred to a neurological unit in an acute confusional state. These are the results of CSF examination:

Protein	0.46 g/l
White cell count	$< 5/mm^3$
Glucose	2.4 mmol/l
	(Blood glucose 5.8 mmol/l)
TPHA	Positive
VDRL	Negative

How would you interpret these findings?

Question 12

The table below shows the results of upper limb nerve conduction studies performed on a 40 year old woman complaining of intermittent 'pins and needles' in the fingers of both hands which often waken her from sleep. Lower limb nerve conduction studies were entirely normal.

	Right	Left	Normal range
Median motor conduction			
Latency [wrist – abductor pollicis brevis (APB)]	4.6	5.7	< 4.4 ms
Amplitude (wrist – APB)	9.1	7.5	> 4.2 mV
Amplitude (cubital fossa – APB)	7.7	4.6	> 4.2 mV
Conduction velocity (wrist – cubital fossa)	55.0	53.8	> 49 m/s
Ulnar motor conduction			
Latency [wrist – abductor digiti minimi (ADM)]	3.0		< 3.5 ms
Amplitude (wrist – ADM)	10.5		> 5.6 mV
Amplitude (below epicondyle – ADM)	8.4		> 5.6 mV
Amplitude (above epicondyle – ADM)	8.8		> 5.6 mV
Conduction velocity (below epicondyle – wrist)	61.0		> 49 m/s
Conduction velocity (above epicondyle – wrist)	64.0		> 49 m/s
Median sensory conduction			
Latency (wrist – palm)	3.4	4.7	< 2.2 ms
Amplitude (wrist – palm)	36.1	15.0	> 40 μV
Ulnar sensory conduction			
Latency (wrist – palm)	2.1	2.0	< 2.2 ms
Amplitude (wrist – palm)	18.0	23.9	> 15 μV

(a) How would you interpret these findings?
(b) What is the definitive treatment?

Question 13

The haematological profile of a 20 year old man presenting with headache, papilloedema and ataxia is shown below.

White blood count	$6.2 \times 10^9/l$
Red blood count	$8.2 \times 10^{12}/l$
Haemoglobin	19.9 g/dl
Haematocrit	57
MCV	91 fl
MCH	31.5 pg
MCHC	35.0 g/dl
Platelets	$540 \times 10^9/l$

How are the neurological symptoms and haematological abnormalities related?

Question 14

A 25 year old Chinese man was investigated for episodic limb weakness. While symptomatic, biochemical analyses revealed the following results.

Sodium	137 mmol/l
Potassium	2.1 mmol/l
Urea	4.7 mmol/l
Creatinine	92 µmol/l
Calcium	2.41 mmol/l
Phosphate	0.91 mmol/l
Bilirubin	16 mmol/l
AST	39 IU/l
ALT	34 IU/l
Alkaline phosphatase	104 IU/l
Albumin	42 g/l
Globulin	27 g/l
Free T4	47 pmol/l

What is the diagnosis?

Question 15

A 21 year old woman developed an acute illness comprising chorea, fever and altered behaviour. She had no significant medical or family history, and was taking no drugs. There were no cardiac signs and neurological examination was otherwise normal. Investigations revealed the following results.

ESR	56 mm in the first hour
Haemoglobin	10.1 g/dl
White count	$2.8 \times 10^9/l$ (55% lymphocytes, 42% neutrophils)
Platelets	$100 \times 10^9/l$
Urea	7.2 mmol/l
Creatinine	116 µmol/l
Sodium	137 mmol/l
Potassium	4.2 mmol/l
Bilirubin	17 µmol/l
AST	92 IU/l
ALT	81 IU/l
GGT	68 IU/l
Calcium	2.24 mmol/l
Free T4	16 pmol/l
TSH	2.4 IU/l

(a) Suggest an explanation for these findings.
(b) Which three tests should be performed?

Question 16

A 51 year old dentist was referred because of a 6-month history of gait difficulty. Examination revealed a mild spastic paraparesis, impaired joint position sense at the hallux, absent vibration sense below the medial malleoli and a mildly ataxic gait. The following results were obtained.

White cell count	$5.0 \times 10^9/l$
Haemoglobin	12.2 g/dl
MCV	108 fl
MCH	33.2 pg
MCHC	34.6 g/dl
Platelets	$267 \times 10^9/l$
Serum B12	316 ng/l
Red cell folate	426 µg/l

Antigastric parietal cell antibody	Positive
Anti-intrinsic factor antibody	Negative
Schilling test	Normal

What is the diagnosis?

Question 17

A 40 year old alcoholic presented with a 3-week history of headache, lethargy and mental symptoms. On examination, he was conscious but confused with signs of mild meningeal irritation. Results of CSF examination were as follows.

Pressure	32 cm H_2O
White cells	225/mm^3 (70% lymphocytes, 30% polymorphs)
Protein	1.3 g/l
Glucose	1.7 mmol/l
	(Blood glucose 6.4 mmol/l)
Gram stain	Negative

(a) Which other tests should be conducted on this CSF sample?
(b) What is the most likely diagnosis?

Question 18

A 39 year old woman was admitted into hospital in a semicomatose state. She exhibited multifocal myoclonus but no focal deficit. In the previous 12 months she had experienced two unexplained confusional episodes which resolved within 24 hours. Urea and electrolytes, glucose, calcium and liver function tests were normal. The results of further investigations are shown below.

CT brain	Normal
EEG	Diffusely slow background
	No focal abnormality
CSF	White cells < 5/mm^3
Protein	0.6 g/l
Glucose	2.9 mmol/l
(Blood glucose	5.9 mmol/l)
Free T4	12.6 pmol/l
TSH	2.1 mU/l
Antithyroid microsomal antibody	1:102 400
Antithyroglobulin antibody	Negative

(a) What is the diagnosis?
(b) What treatment is indicated?

Question 19

A previously healthy 48 year old man was admitted with a 2-day history of headache, fever, increasing confusion and seizures. He was taking ampicillin for a sore throat. The first CSF sample was taken on admission and the second sample was obtained 10 days later because of failure to respond to antibiotics and antituberculous chemotherapy.

	First sample	Second sample
White cells	$67/\text{mm}^3$	$150/\text{mm}^3$
Neutrophils	80%	10%
Lymphocytes	20%	90%
Red cells	$1/\text{mm}^3$	$10/\text{mm}^3$
Protein	0.47 g/l	1.2 g/l
CSF glucose	3.8 mmol/l	2.9 mmol/l
Blood glucose	5.6 mmol/l	5.9 mmol/l

What is the likeliest diagnosis?

Question 20

These are the constituents of CSF, obtained at myelography, from a woman with a mild spastic paraparesis, sphincter disturbance and a patchy sensory loss in her legs.

Appearance	Xanthochromic
Red cell count	$2000/\text{mm}^3$
White cell count	$5/\text{mm}^3$
Protein	9.4 g/l
Glucose	3.4 mmol/l
(Blood glucose	6.2 mmol/l)

(a) What is the name for this combination of findings?
(b) How does this occur?

Answer 1

(a) Complete heart block
(b) Insert a permanent pacemaker.
     Stop antiepileptic drugs.

Comment

The attacks are difficult to characterize with any certainty but the light-headedness and profound pallor suggest postural hypotension. In someone of this age cardiac causes of syncope should be excluded. The EEG, itself, reveals muscle artefact on a normal background. However, the electrocardiogram (ECG) lead reveals an 8-second period of complete heart block. The antiepileptic drug was stopped and his attacks ceased after the insertion of a permanent pacemaker.

Answer 2

(a) 3 cycles per second generalized spike and wave (3 cps GSW)
(b) Ethosuximide.

Comment

The EEG reveals a normal background rhythm punctuated by a sudden onset of 3 cps GSW occurring simultaneously across all the leads. The episode lasts for 11 seconds and the EEG abruptly returns to normal. The clinical correlate is a typical absence seizure: sudden onset of loss of consciousness, staring with or without minor motor phenomena, e.g. blinking, of brief duration with rapid recovery of consciousness. This is the only form of seizure which can be labelled 'petit mal' and this is the characteristic seizure type of childhood absence epilepsy. Whilst sodium valproate and the novel antiepileptic drug, lamotrigine, are effective against a wide range of seizure types, ethosuximide is a pure antiabsence drug. Childhood absence epilepsy remits at puberty in approximately 75% of cases.

Answer 3

Acute viral myositis with rhabdomyolysis resulting in acute renal failure.

Comment

The clinical presentation is that of a severe acute proximal myopathy, probably of viral aetiology. The marked elevation of CPK (and transaminases) confirms the presence of rhabdomyolysis. Acute renal failure occurs because of the blockage of the renal tubules by myoglobin. If the acute renal failure is successfully treated, the prognosis for neurological recovery is favourable.

Answer 4

Cryptococcus neuformans.

Comment

This man has an aseptic meningitis: fever, headache, other signs of meningeal irritation, and a predominantly lymphocytic pleocytosis with normal CSF glucose. In the majority of cases where a cause is identified, the aetiology is viral. However, the presence of immunosuppression (HIV positive) demands exclusion of more sinister conditions. HIV itself can cause aseptic meningitis but seroconversion occurs during convalescence. Acute neurosyphilis may present in this way but is effectively excluded by the negative serology. While tuberculous meningitis can be remarkably insidious, the conscious level is usually depressed, CSF protein markedly elevated and CSF glucose markedly diminished.

Cryptococcal meningitis is the most frequent fungal complication of HIV infection. It causes a subacute granulomatous meningitis. Presentations include a severe meningoencephalitis, raised intracranial pressure and focal deficits, but the onset can be remarkably indolent and the diagnosis should be considered in any immunocompromised individual even in the absence of systemic upset or neurological signs. Small numbers of organisms are found in the CSF and, therefore, large volumes are required to facilitate diagnostic testing. Indian ink staining is positive in 50–60% of cases. A negative latex agglutination test excludes the diagnosis with 95% probability. Intravenous amphotericin is the treatment of choice but mortality is 40% even in the absence of immunosuppression.

Answer 5

(a) Chronic inflammatory demyelinating polyneuropathy (CIDP).
(b) Oral prednisolone.

Comment

This condition, sometimes called chronic Guillain–Barré syndrome (GBS), can be distinguished from acute GBS on clinical and neurophysiological grounds.

Acute GBS, a purely motor demyelinating neuropathy, can be diagnosed only if the duration of symptoms is less than 6 weeks. CIDP is manifest by gradual progression of symptoms over several months. Motor features predominate but sensory symptoms and signs are common. In both conditions CSF examination reveals raised protein but no cells. Neurophysiological testing reveals evidence of demyelination; acute GBS is characterized by markedly delayed motor nerve conduction velocities (NCVs), while CIDP produces mild to moderate delay of both motor and sensory nerve conduction. Recognition of CIDP is important because 90% of patients respond to high-dose oral prednisolone. In those who fail to respond or, indeed, in the 10–15% who subsequently relapse, plasma exchange or intravenous immunogloblins are usually effective.

Answer 6

(a) Polymyositis.
(b) Serum creatinine phosphokinase and gamma glutamyl transferase.
(c) Prednisolone with or without azathioprine.

Comment

This woman presented with a subacute weakness of proximal limb muscles without evidence of dermatitis or connective tissue disease. While elevated transaminases (AST, ALT) occur in both liver and muscle disease, GGT and CPK are specific liver and muscle enzymes, respectively. The diagnosis of idiopathic polymyositis was confirmed by muscle biopsy which revealed widespread segmental necrosis of muscle fibres, myophagia, evidence of regeneration and infiltration of inflammatory cells. Treatment involves either prednisolone alone or a combination of prednisolone and azathioprine. Remission of symptoms usually occurs permitting a cautious reduction of immunosuppressive therapy. However, complete recovery occurs in only 20–25% of cases. Occult malignancy occurs less commonly than in patients with dermatomyositis. However, like dermatomyositis, polymyositis often antedates the clinical manifestations of malignancy.

Answer 7

(a) Generalized periodic sharp wave complexes.
(b) Creutzfeldt–Jacob disease.

Comment

The clinical picture suggests a rapidly progressive dementia with cortical blindness. The 16-channel EEG (top eight channels –right hemisphere) reveals a generally slow background rhythm, particularly on the left, with several generalized periodic sharp wave complexes appearances which are typical of established CJD.

Answer 8

Free T3.

Comment

The clinical presentation (weight loss, tremor, heart failure, proximal myopathy) is highly suggestive of thyrotoxicosis. This woman's free T3 level was 70.3 pmol/l (NR 2.0–5.5 pmol/l) in the presence of normal free T4 levels. T3 toxicosis accounts for approximately 10% of 'thyrotoxicosis'.

Slowly progressive proximal muscle weakness is common in untreated hyperthyroidism. The severity of weakness correlates poorly with the level of thyroid hormone. Serum CPK is usually normal, although rhabdomyolysis may occur in 'thyroid storm'. EMG usually reveals myopathic changes (brief, low amplitude, polyphasic motor unit potentials with or without fibrillations/fasciculations), while repetitive motor nerve stimulation may reveal evidence of abnormal neuromuscular transmission. Muscle biopsy is normal or reveals occasional small necrotic fibres. Symptoms may improve with propranalol and resolve completely when a euthyroid state is reached.

Answer 9

Evidence of previous right optic nerve demyelination supporting a diagnosis of multiple sclerosis.

Comment

A visual evoked response is produced by a sudden change of a viewed chequer board (pattern-shift visual evoked response, PSVER). This permits detection of conductional delays in visual pathways in patients who had previously suffered disease of the optic nerves (symptomatic or subclinical) even in the absence of residual clinical evidence thereof (pale optic disc, relative afferent pupillary defect). Unilateral prolongation of latency indicates involvement of one optic nerve while bilateral delay implies bilateral optic nerve disease or a postchiasmal lesion. Demyelination is the commonest pathology but similar findings can be seen in toxic or nutritional amblyopia, ischaemic optic neuropathy or Leber's hereditary optic neuropathy. The finding of an abnormal PSVER in someone with a clinically apparent lesion elsewhere within the CNS is presumptive evidence of MS. It should be emphasized that MRI of brain has superseded visual evoked responses (VERs) in the investigation of patients with possible MS.

Answer 10

(a) Reye's syndrome
(b) Blood ammonia level.

Comment

In a child presenting with fever and coma, the presence of a metabolic acidosis, hypoglycaemia, raised transaminases and markedly elevated blood ammonia level are characteristic of Reye's syndrome. Outbreaks have been associated with various viral infections and sporadic cases attributed to aspirin. Pathologically there is cerebral oedema and fatty infiltration of the viscera, especially the liver. Once coma occurs the mortality rate is 50–60%, but early diagnosis and supportive therapy have reduced mortality to approximately 10%.

Answer 11

Previously treated neurosyphilis.

Comment

The presence of specific antitreponemal antibodies in an otherwise normal CSF (protein, cells, negative VDRL) is evidence of previous, probably treated, neurosyphilis. Whilst the specific tests [TPHA, fluorescent treponemal antibody (FTA-abs)] are useful in establishing the diagnosis, the non-specific tests (e.g. VDRL) are used to assess disease activity and response to treatment. In this case, the CSF findings were unrelated to the clinical presentation.

Answer 12

(a) Bilateral (left worse than right) carpal tunnel syndrome.
(b) Carpal tunnel decompression.

Comment

Paraesthesiae which waken a patient at night or which are triggered by gripping suggest median nerve compression at the wrist. This is often associated with local wrist pain which may be referred to the forearm, elbow, upper arm or shoulder. On examination the classical $3\frac{1}{2}$ digit (thumb, index, middle, half of ring) sensory loss is rarely observed. Most commonly there is impaired sensation over the palmar aspect of the thumb and the tips of the other fingers. Confirmation of the diagnosis by nerve conduction studies is essential because other causes (median nerve compression in the forearm, median neuropathy as part of a more widespread neuropathy) will not respond to surgical treatment. Reversible causes of carpal tunnel syndrome, e.g. hypothyroidism or pregnancy should also be excluded. In this case there is bilaterally increased distal median motor and sensory latencies with normal forearm conduction velocities, and normal ulnar motor and sensory nerve conduction. Wrist splints worn overnight can produce symptomatic benefit and steroid injection into the carpal tunnel may cause temporarily relief but surgical decompression of the median nerves is the definitive treatment.

Answer 13

Cerebellar haemangioblastoma.

Comment

These lesions present with raised intracranial pressure, unilateral cerebellar signs with or without unilateral/bilateral pyramidal signs or involvement of the 5th–8th cranial nerves. In large series, secondary polycythaemia, presumably due to secretion of erythropoetin by the tumour, occurs in approximately 15% of cases. Surgical excision is curative but local recurrence is well recognized. Furthermore, the index case should be thoroughly investigated for evidence of multiple haemangiomata (Von Hippel–Lindau disease), the implications of which are discussed in Grey Case 32.

Answer 14

Hypokalaemic periodic paralysis secondary to hyperthyroidism.

Comment

Disorders of muscle excitability are caused by defects in genes encoding muscle ion channels. Hyperkalaemic and hypokalaemic periodic paralysis, which are often clinically difficult to distinguish, are due to defects of sodium and calcium channels, respectively. Hypokalaemic periodic paralysis has been linked to a region of Clq (long arm of chromosome 1) encoding the alpha 1 subunit of L-type calcium channels. However, the relationship between the inactivation of this channel and hypokalaemia-induced attacks of muscle weakness is not fully understood.

Approximately 10% of oriental patients with thyrotoxicosis suffer this complication. Acute symptoms respond to potassium supplements and further attacks can be prevented by treatment of the thyrotoxicosis. In primary hypokalaemic periodic paralysis, carbonic anhydrase inhibitors, e.g. acetazolamide may be effective.

Answer 15

(a) Systemic lupus erythematosus.
(b) Antidouble-stranded DNA antibody;
    Pregnancy test;
    Copper studies.

Comment

In this context, the raised ESR, neutropenia and thrombocytopenia are highly suggestive of SLE. Chorea occurs in only 2% of patients with SLE but it can be the sole presenting feature.

Chorea gravidarum should be considered. Whilst the negative past medical history and normal cardiac examination virtually exclude this cause, a pregnancy test is indicated. The mildly deranged liver function tests (LFTs) demand that copper studies be performed, since Wilson's disease, whilst extremely unlikely, should be excluded because it is treatable. Even in the absence of a positive family history, Huntington's disease should be considered but DNA testing is not indicated when an alternative diagnosis is more likely.

Other metabolic causes of chorea (hypoglycaemia, hypernatraemia, hypocalcaemia, thyrotoxicosis) are all excluded by the normal tests.

Answer 16

Chronic nitrous oxide intoxication.

Comment

The physical findings of pyramidal weakness and impaired dorsal column sensation suggest subacute combined degeneration of the cord. Whilst he has a peripheral macrocytosis, the normal serum B12, red cell folate and Schilling test exclude malabsorption and pernicious anaemia, respectively. Chronic 'recreational use' of nitrous oxide causes an identical clinical picture, possibly because nitrous oxide interferes with B12 utilization. Cessation of exposure results in complete relief of symptoms.

Answer 17

(a) Ziehl–Nielson stain;
    Latex agglutination tests for bacterial antigens;
    Culture for pyogenic organisms, tubercle bacilli and fungi.
(b) Tuberculous meningitis.

Comment

The insidious onset, mild meningeal irritation and CSF reaction make pyogenic meningitis unlikely, but cultures are essential. The clinical features and CSF findings (predominantly lymphocytic pleocytosis, high protein and low sugar) of tuberculous and fungal meningitis are virtually indistinguishable. A chest X-ray to exclude or identify evidence of pulmonary tuberculosis is required. On the grounds of probability, alcoholics are much more likely to contract tuberculous meningitis and most patients with fungal meningitis are immunocompromised. This patient should receive broad-spectrum antibiotics and antituberculous chemotherapy until culture results are obtained.

Answer 18

(a) Hashimoto's encephalopathy.
(b) High-dose oral steroids.

Comment

While rare, Hashimoto's encephalopathy is probably underdiagnosed and thyroid autoantibodies should be requested in anyone with an unexplained 'metabolic encephalopathy'. It presents as a relapsing encephalopathy in patients who are usually euthyroid with high titres of antithyroid autoantibodies. However, cases have been reported in which individuals have been either hypothyroid or hyperthyroid when encephalopathic.

The central feature is depression of consciousness but seizures, focal or generalized, are common, and transient focal deficits may occur. Investigation reveals an 'encephalopathic EEG', raised CSF protein and a normal CT scan. The pathophysiology is unknown, but cerebral vasculitis and autoimmune encephalopathy have been postulated. Most patients respond to steroids but additional immunosuppressive therapy may be required.

Answer 19

Viral encephalitis.

Comment

The presentation and initial CSF sample do not permit distinction between viral encephalitis, partially treated bacterial meningitis and tuberculous meningitis. However, seizures occurring early in the course of the illness, the increasingly lymphocytic CSF with a normal glucose level and a lack of response to treatment favour an encephalitic process, with *Herpes simplex* being the likeliest offending organism. The diagnosis is important because the outcome is directly related to the duration of this condition prior to commencement of antiviral treatment. When in doubt, intravenous acyclovir should be administered.

Answer 20

(a) Froin's syndrome.
(b) CSF block.

Comment

A rise in CSF protein implies pathological processes in or near the ependyma or meninges. Moderate elevations (0.5–2 g/l) are seen in viral encephalitis. Bacterial meningitis, by increasing capillary perfusion in choroidal or meningeal vessels, provokes a greater rise (up to 5 g/l). Similar levels can be seen in tuberculous meningitis and some cases of acute Guillian–Barré syndrome. Levels as high as 10 g/l imply loculation of lumbar CSF owing to blockage of CSF pathways usually by a malignant process. CSF typically appears yellow and clots readily owing to the presence of fibrinogen.

Slide Interpretation

Question 1

This man has a mild degree of learning disability and epilepsy.

(a) What is the skin lesion?
(b) How is the condition inherited?

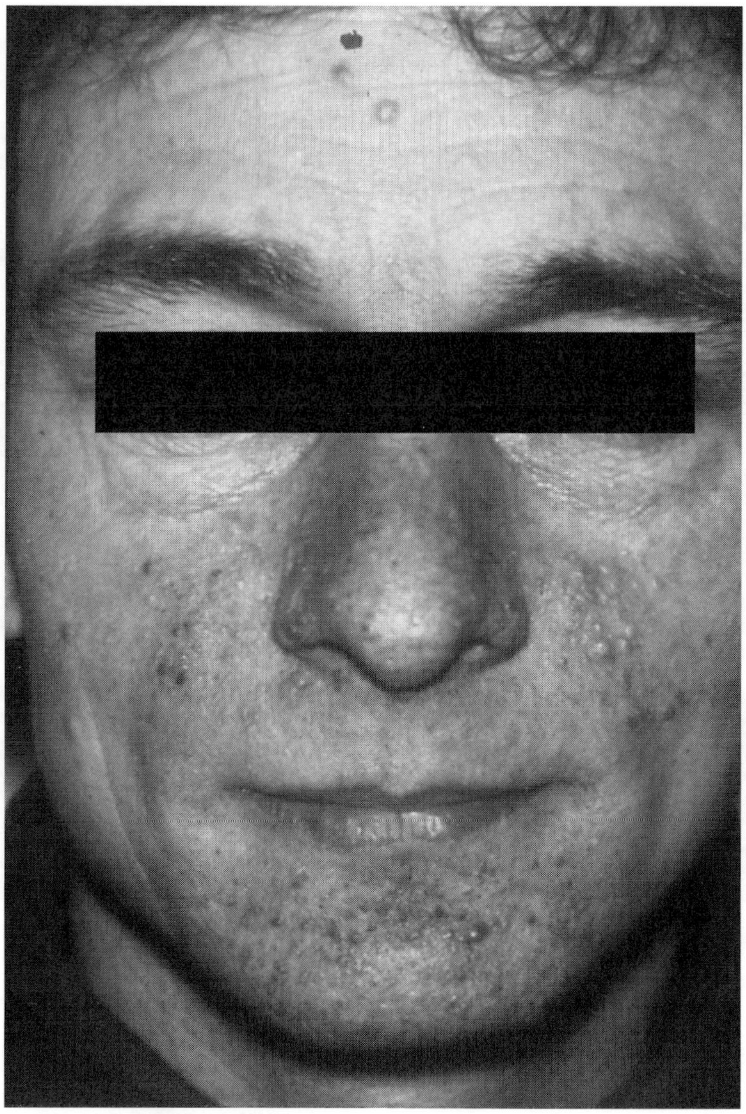

See Slide 1, Colour Plate Section

Question 2

A young man was involved in a road traffic accident.

What does his CT scan show?

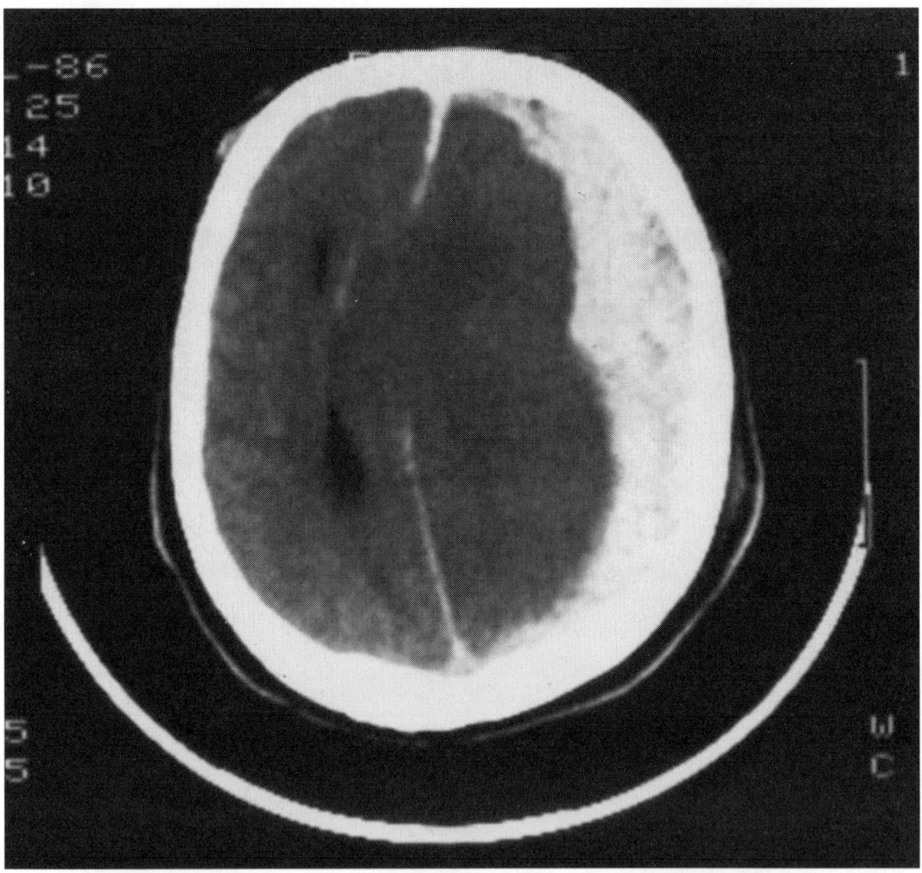

Question 3

(a) What is this radiological sign?
(b) What is the underlying pathology?

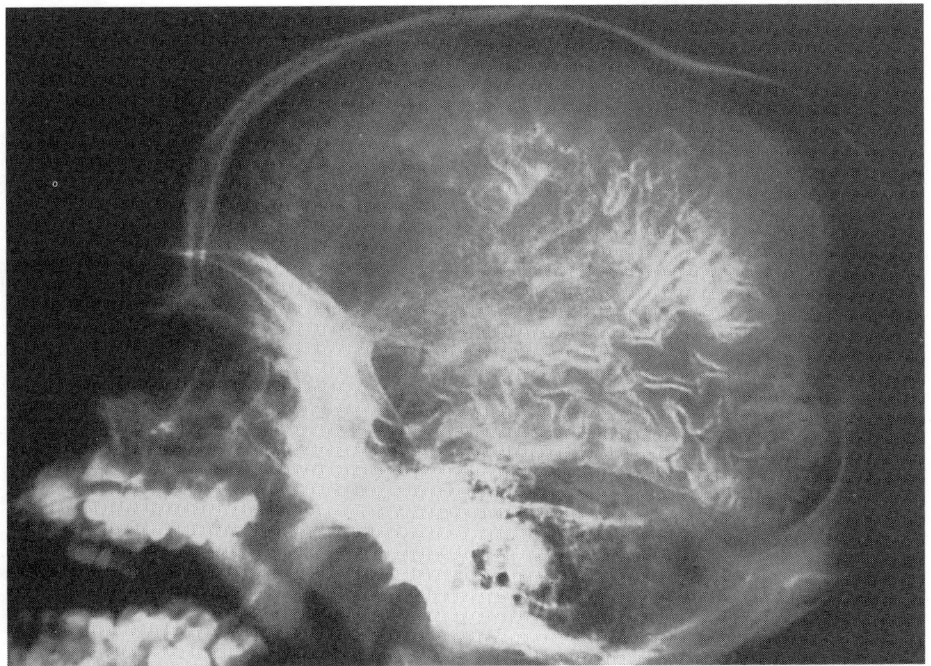

Question 4

A 16 year old boy presented with progressive myoclonic epilepsy, muscle weakness and ataxia.

(a) What is demonstrated on the muscle biopsy?
(b) Name the condition.

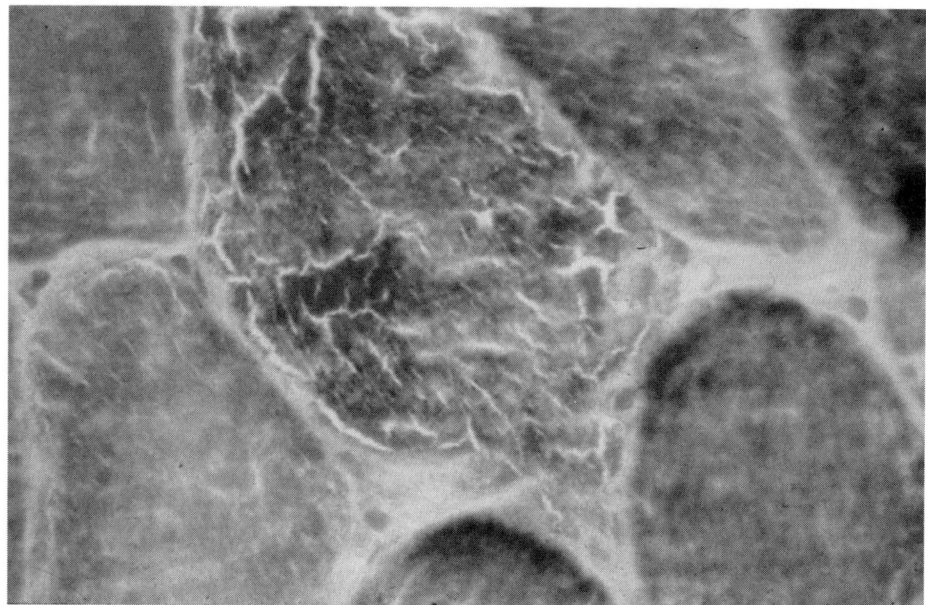

See Slide 2, Colour Plate Section

Question 5

While recovering from gastroenteritis, this man developed weakness of all four limbs, slurred speech and difficulty swallowing.

(a) What does the MRI scan reveal?
(b) What was the likeliest cause?
(c) What is the prognosis?

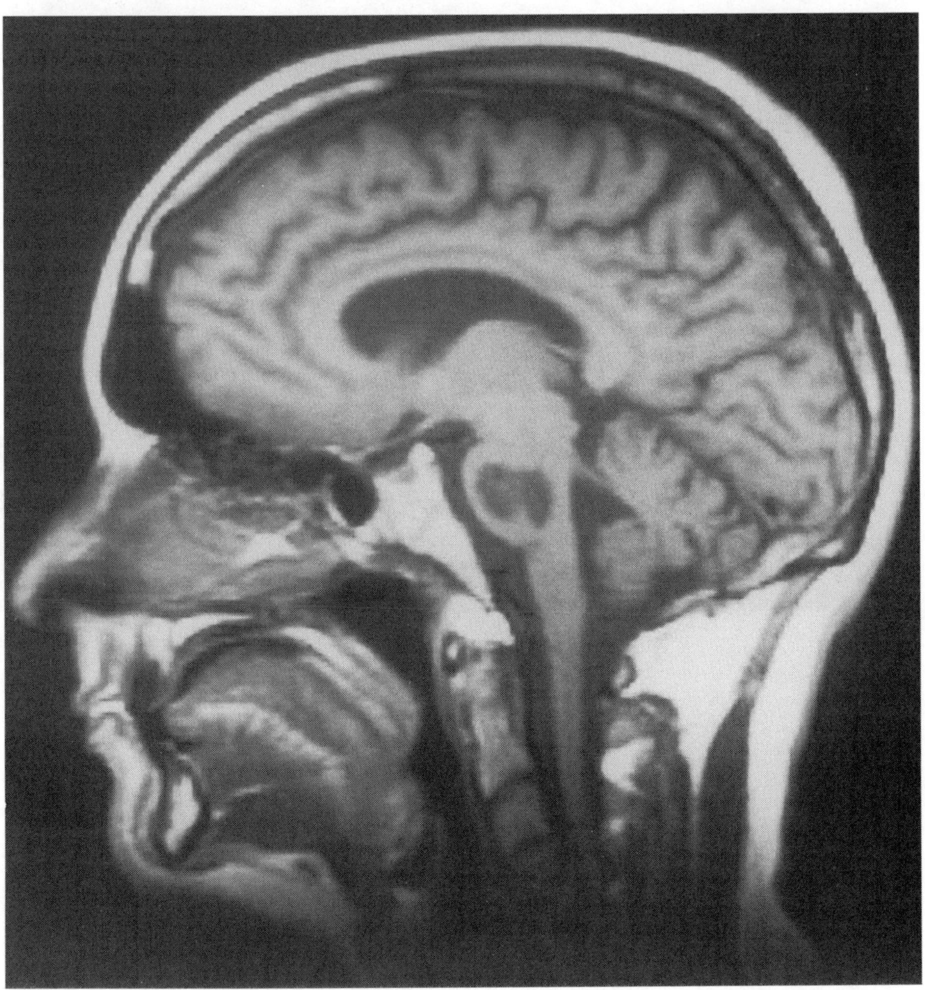

Question 6

This 62 year old woman complained of 'pins and needles' in the tips of her thumb and index finger.

(a) What does the photograph reveal?
(b) What is the likeliest explanation?

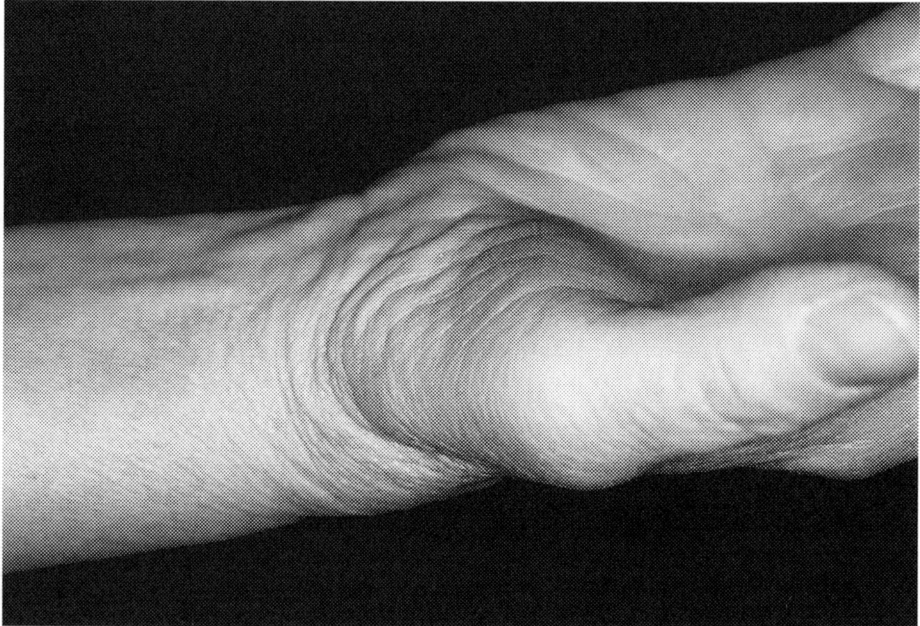

Question 7

Ten years after a successful renal transplant, this woman presented with raised intracranial pressure. CT scans were taken before (above) and after treatment (below).

(a) What is the lesion?
(b) What was the treatment?

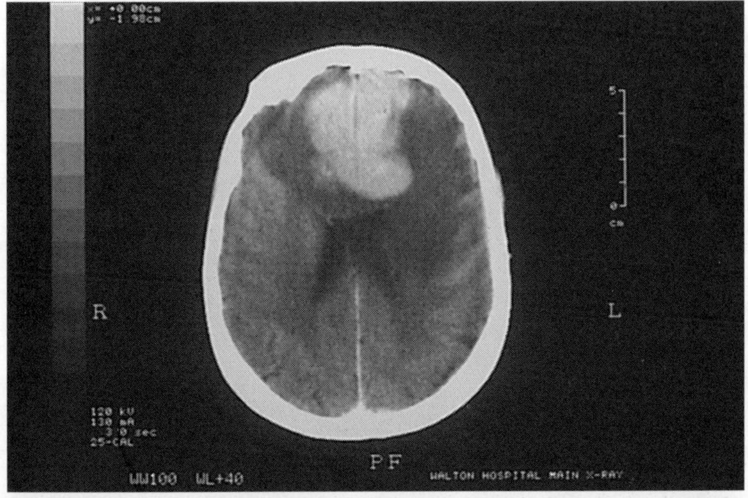

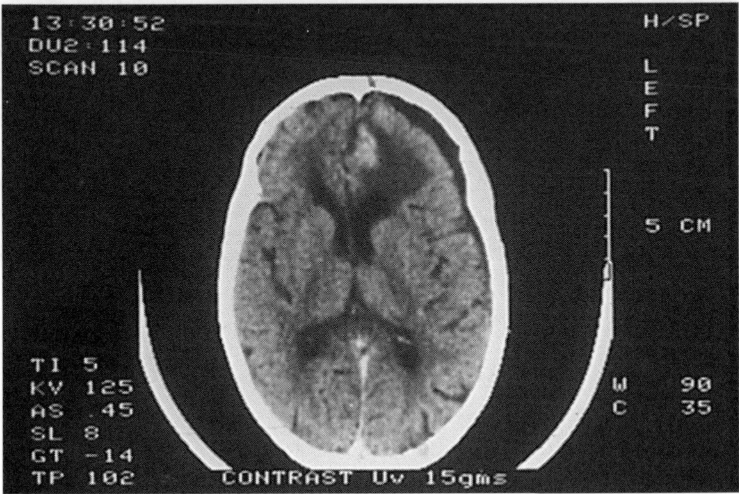

Question 8

This patient reported left-sided deafness.

Which genetically determined condition explains the MR appearances?

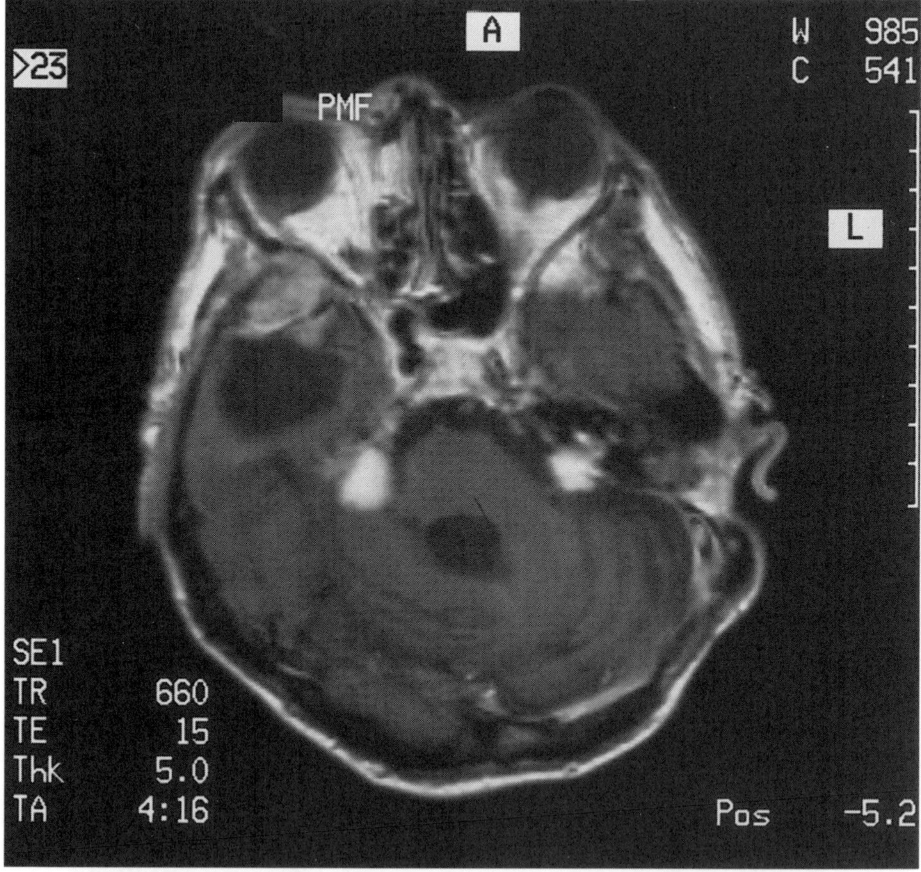

Question 9

These CT scan appearances are characteristic of which condition?

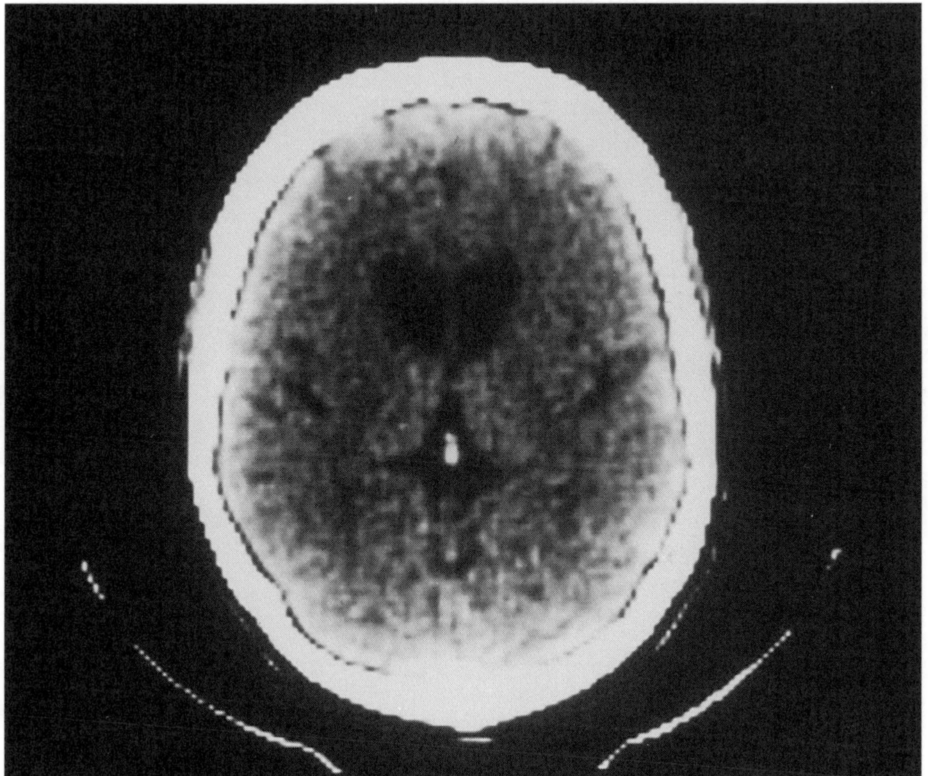

Question 10

This elderly woman is unable to elevate her eyelids (left) or move her eyes in any direction (right).

Name two possible causes of these signs.

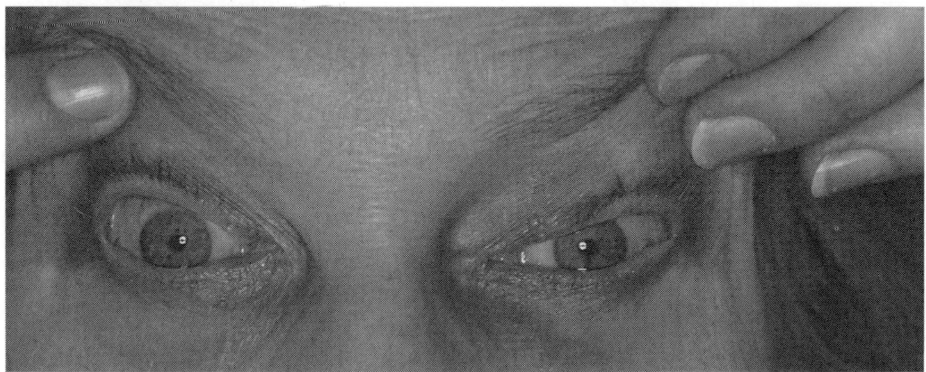

Question 11

Name three causes of this X-ray appearance.

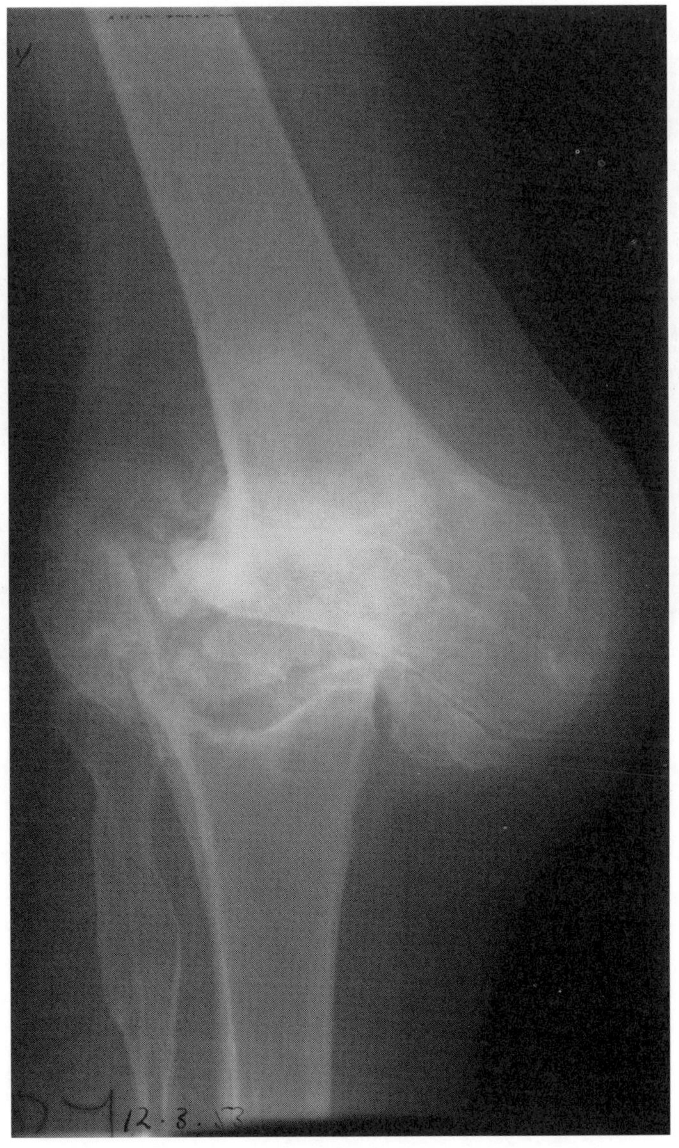

Question 12

How did this man present?

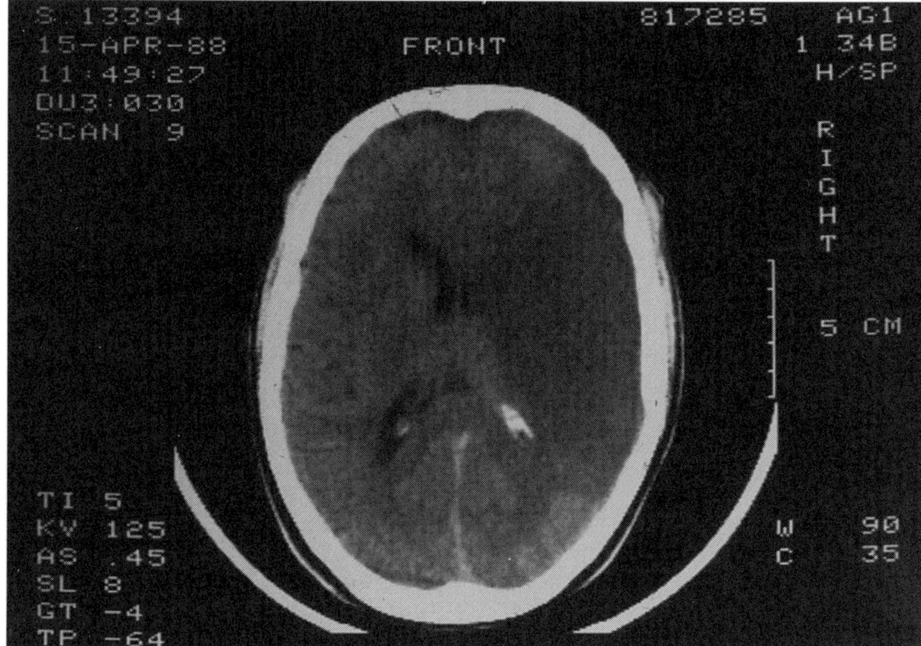

Question 13

Name this clinical sign.

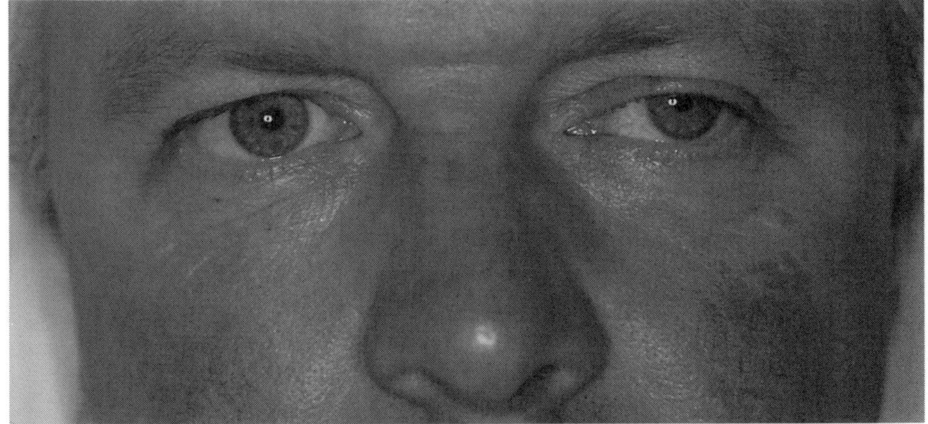

Question 14

This is the magnetic resonance angiogram of the patient depicted in slide 13 on page 105.

What does it show?

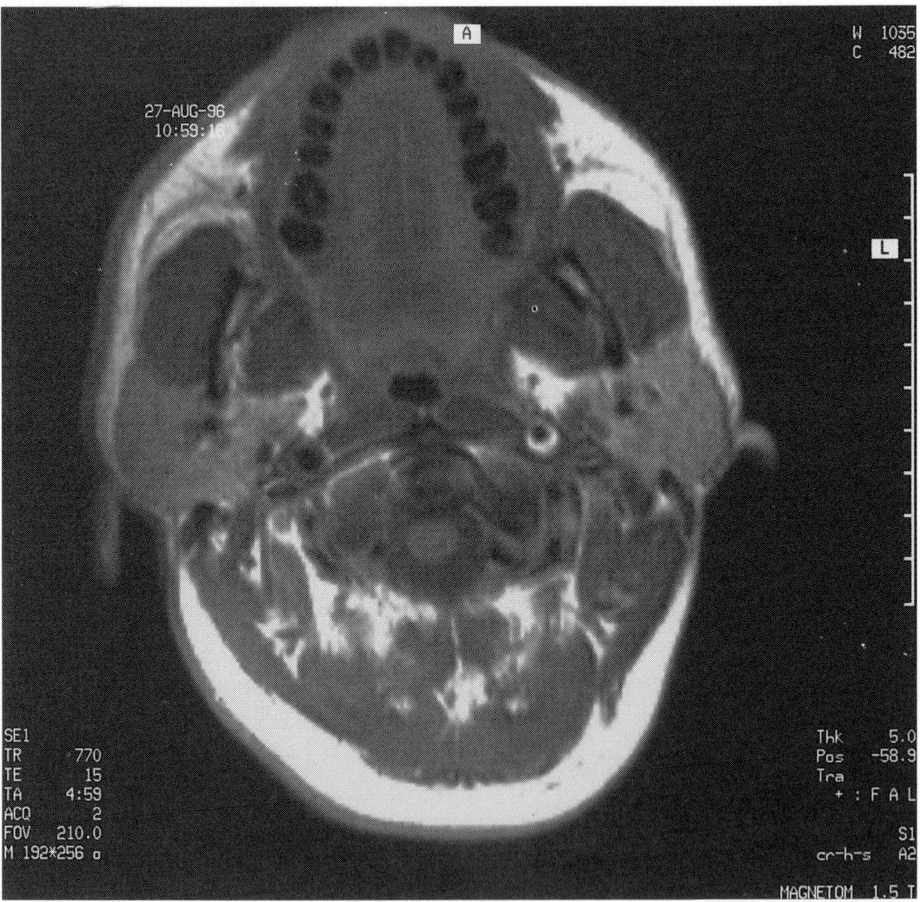

Question 15

What is responsible for this appearance?

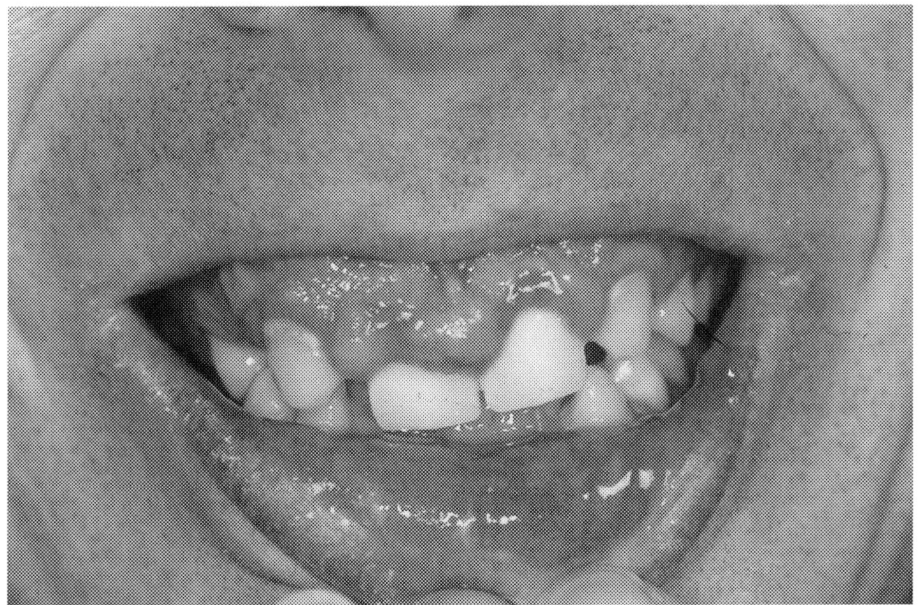

See Slide 3, Colour Plate Section

Question 16

(a) What does this skull X-ray show?
(b) What is the commonest late complication of this insult?

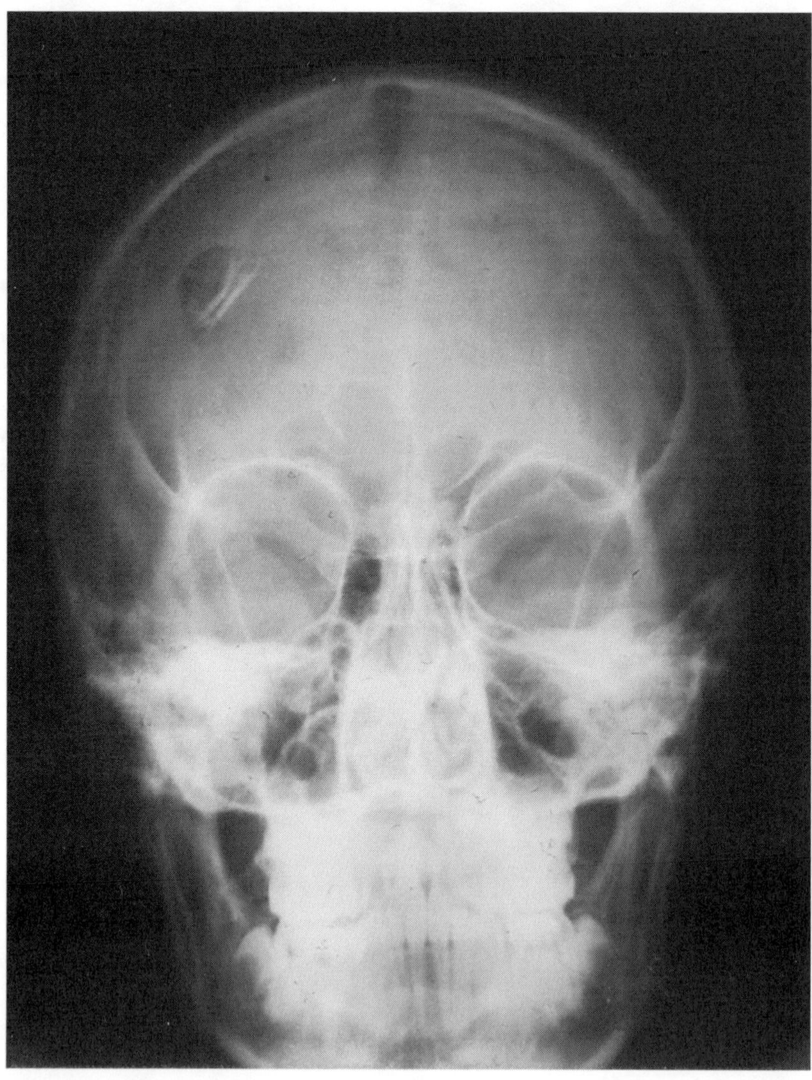

Question 17

What is the cause of this woman's ocular signs?

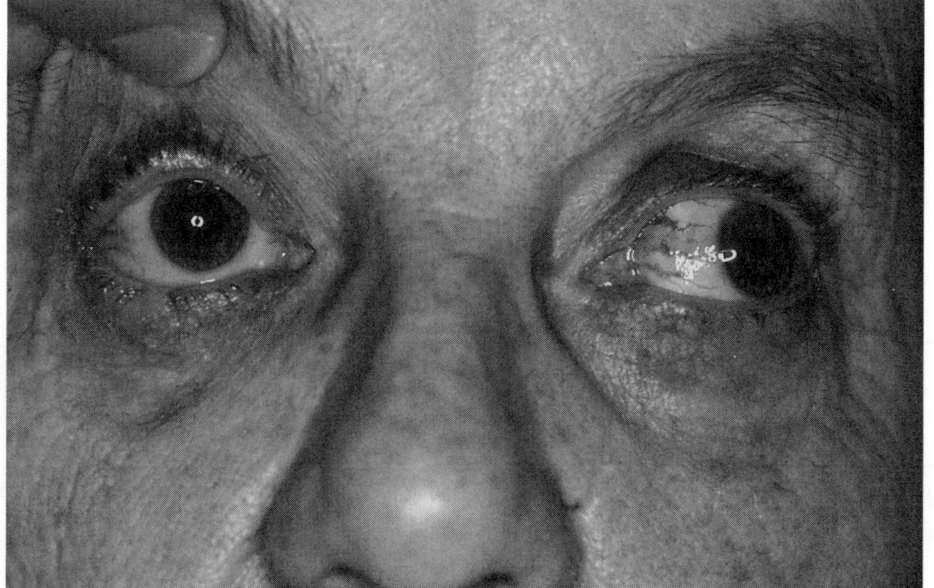

Question 18

Two weeks postpartum, this woman developed acutely raised intracranial pressure.

(a) What does the MRI show?
(b) What is the cause?
(c) How should this be treated?

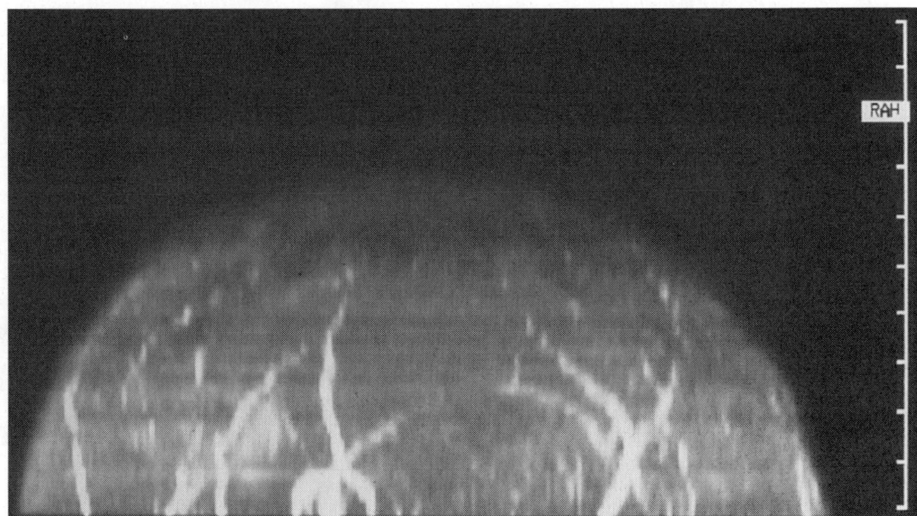

Question 19

Name two possible clinical presentations of this lesion.

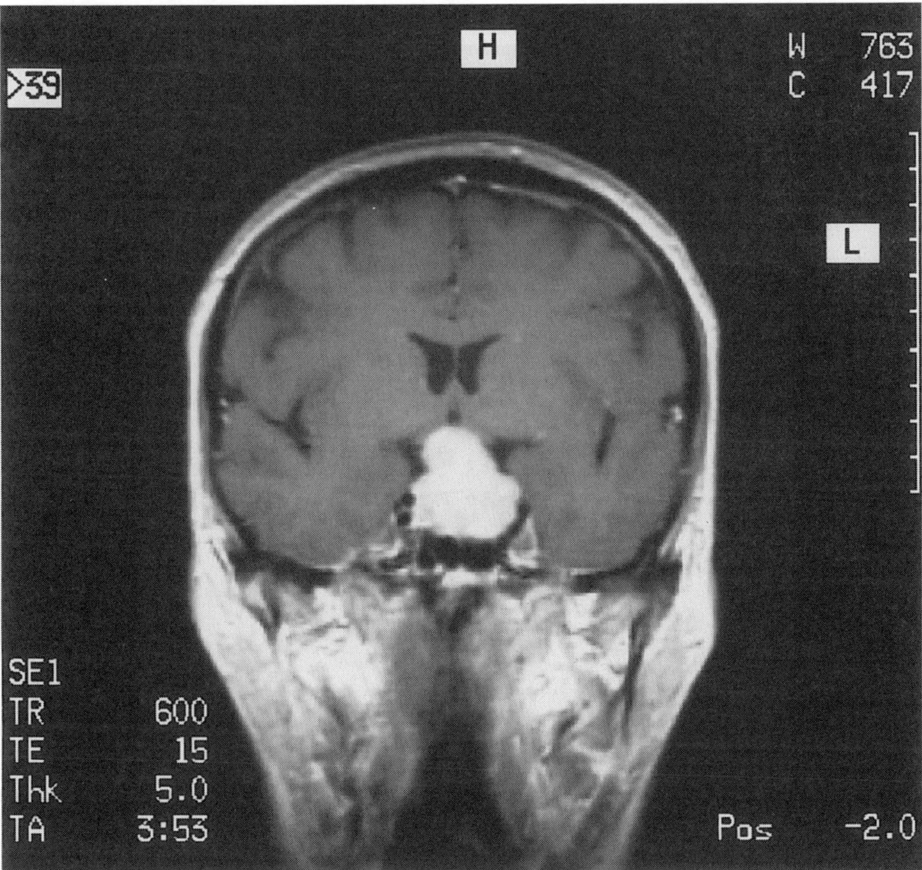

Question 20

(a) What is the name of this angiographic appearance (above)? A normal right carotid angiogram is shown for comparison (below).
(b) What are the clinical presentations thereof?

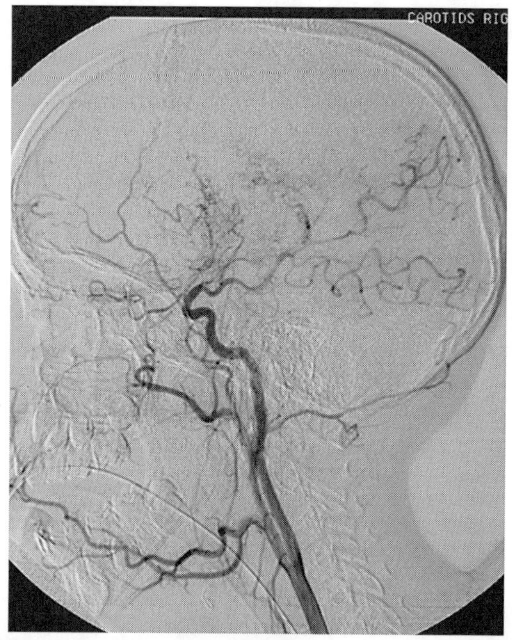

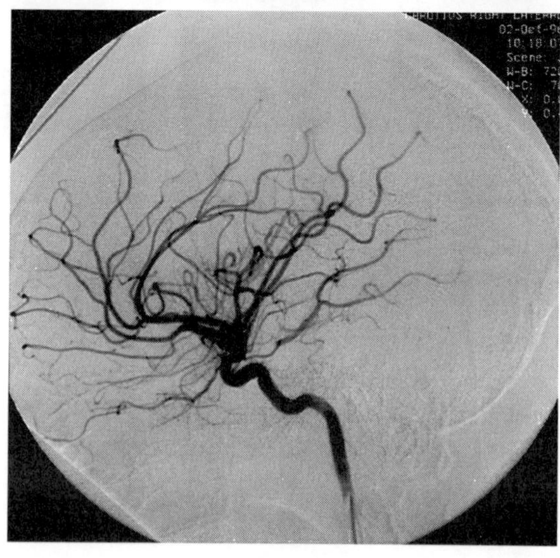

Question 21

A postmortem was performed on a 72 year old man with progressive cognitive decline until death.

Of which condition are the histological appearances indicative?

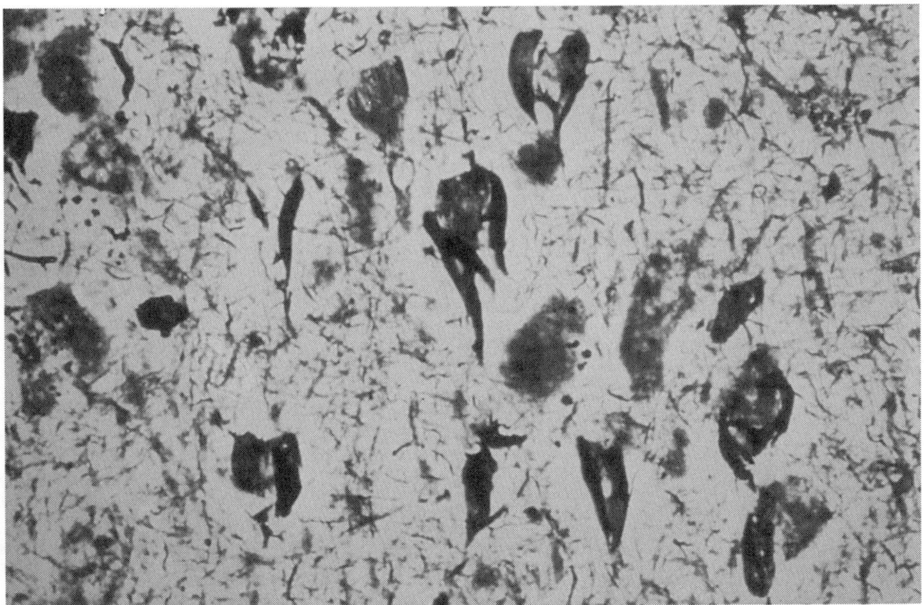

See Slide 4, Colour Plate Section

Question 22

A 35 year old doctor, employed by the World Health Organization, has travelled extensively throughout the Indian subcontinent and South America.

(a) What does his CT scan show?
(b) What is the commonest presentation of this condition?
(c) What other presentations are described?

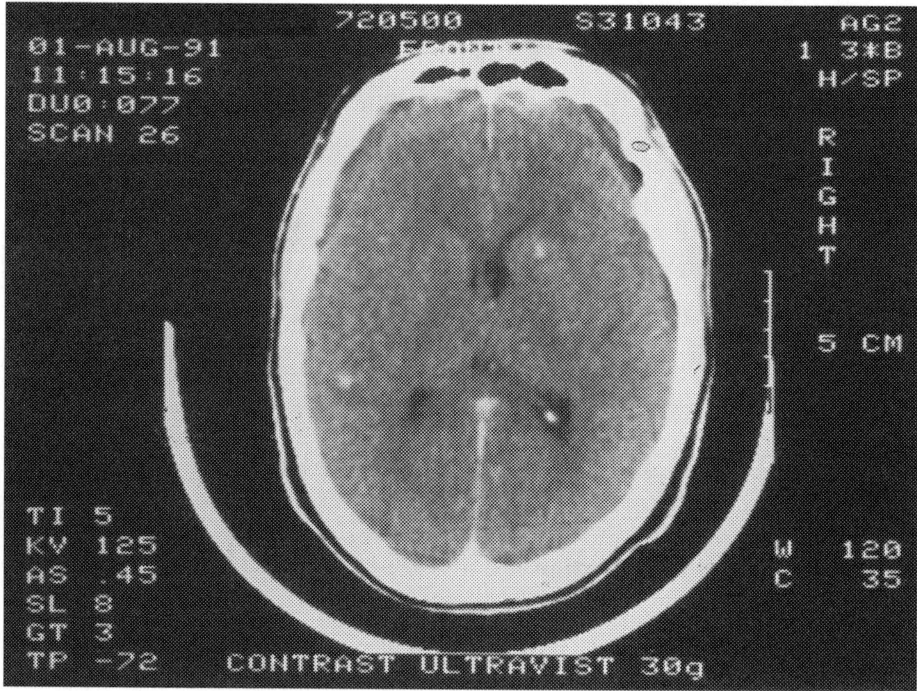

Question 23

This young woman was a front-seat passenger in a car which was involved in a head-on collision.

(a) Name the physical sign.
(b) How might this be explained?

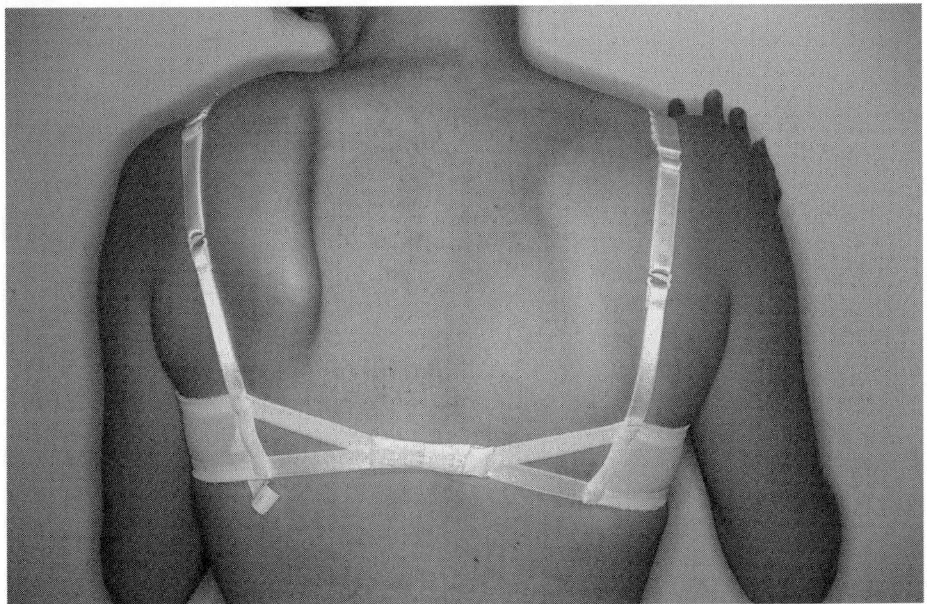

Question 24

(a) Describe the MR appearances.
(b) Name two possible causes.

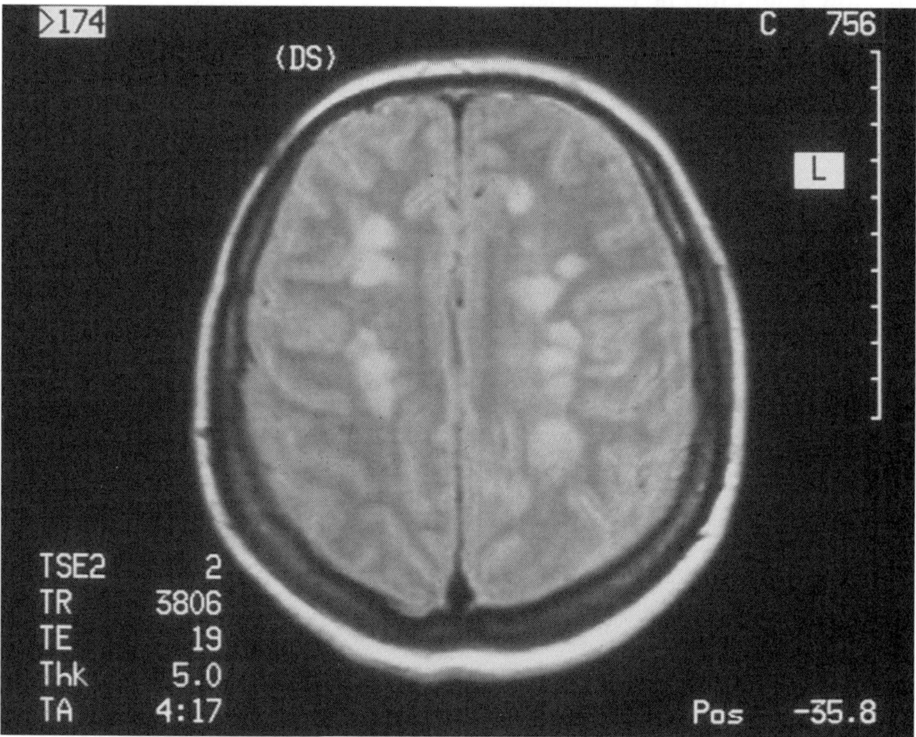

Question 25

(a) What is the angiographic diagnosis (above)? A normal left carotid angiogram is shown for comparison (below).
(b) What is the commonest presentation?

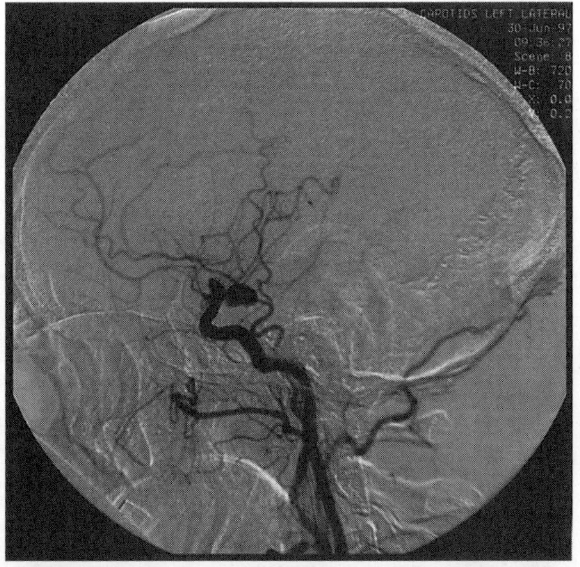

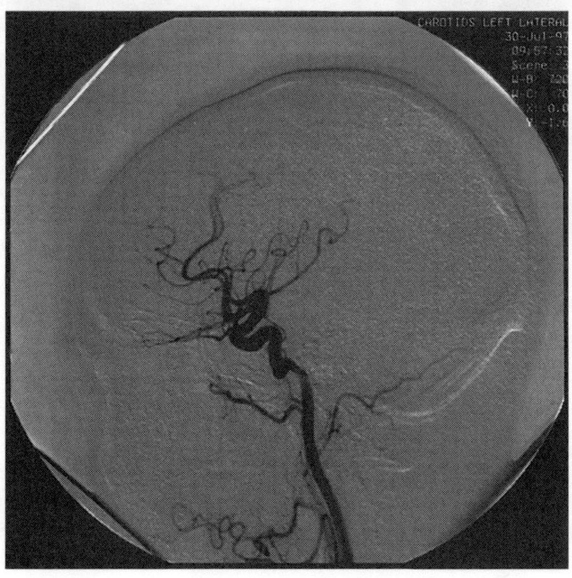

Question 26

These are pre-contrast (above) and post-contrast (below) CT scans of an HIV-positive patient with a right hemiparesis.

(a) What is the likeliest cause?
(b) What treatment is indicated?

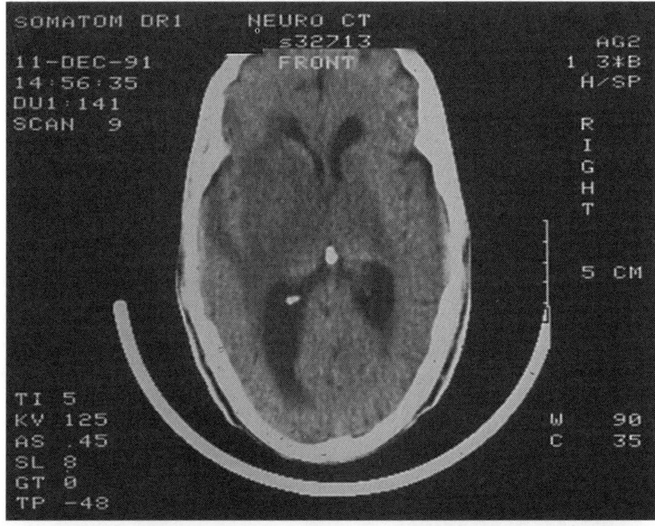

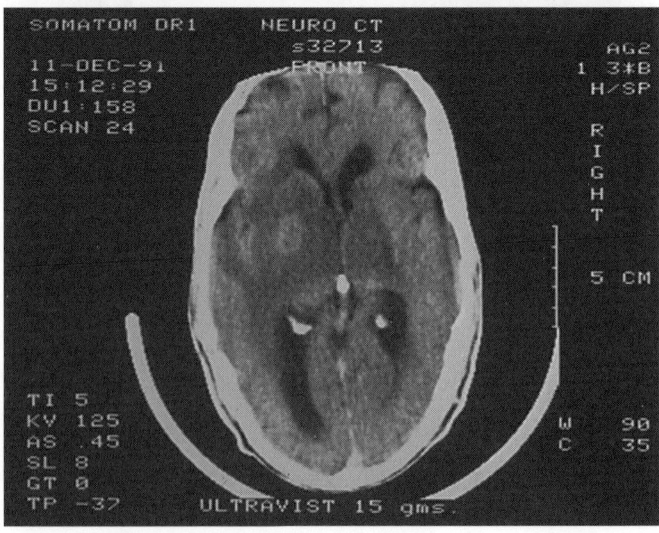

Question 27

(a) Name the physical signs seen on this photograph.
(b) Why did she present to a neurologist?
(c) What is the prognosis of her neurological condition?

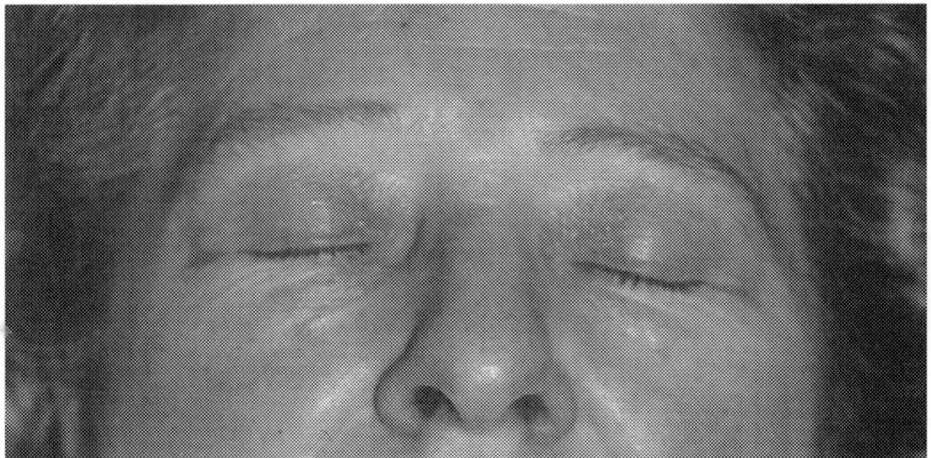

See Slide 5, Colour Plate Section

Question 28

This 54 year old man presented with progressive gait difficulty and slurred speech. Examination revealed ataxia, dysarthria and mild extrapyramidal rigidity.

(a) What does the MRI scan reveal?
(b) What is the prognosis?

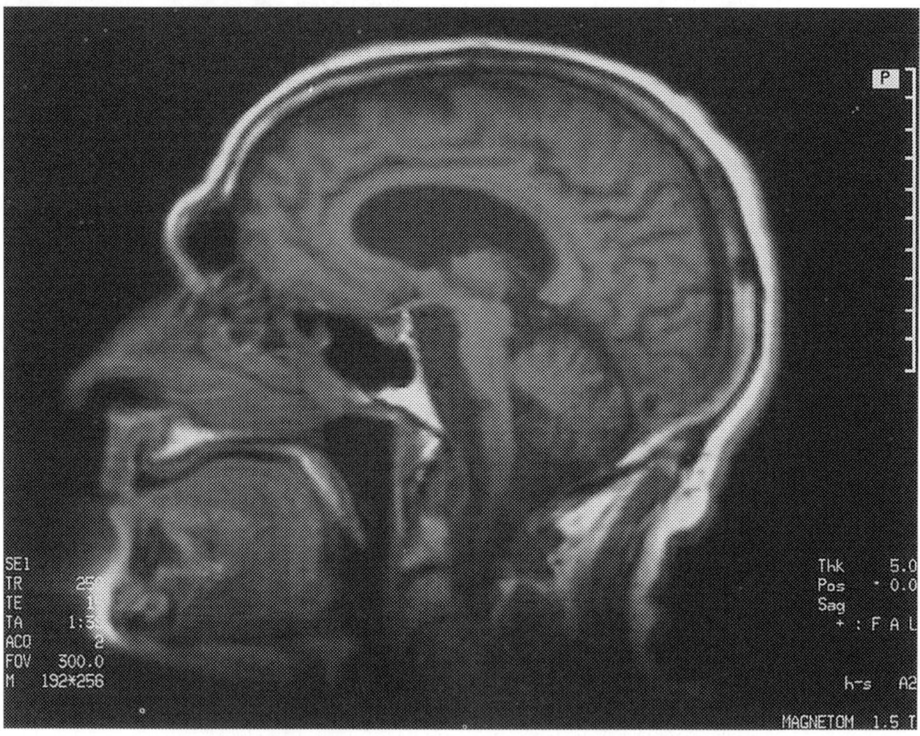

Question 29

(a) What is shown on this cervical myelogram?
(b) What is the likeliest explanation?

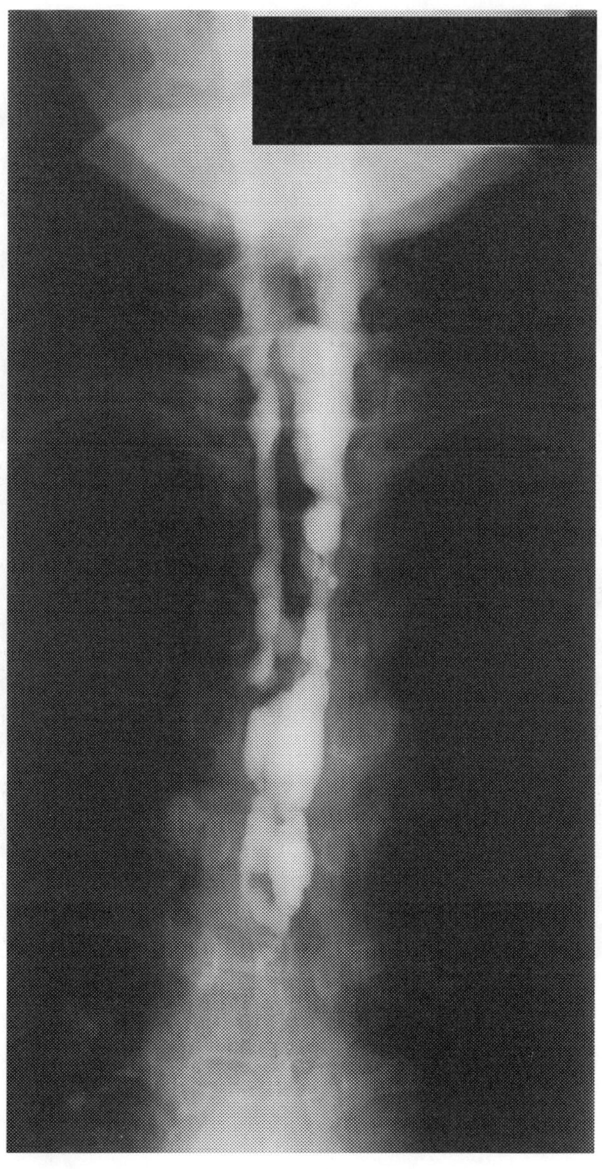

Question 30

(a) What is the lesion shown on CT scan?
(b) Name two possible clinical presentations.

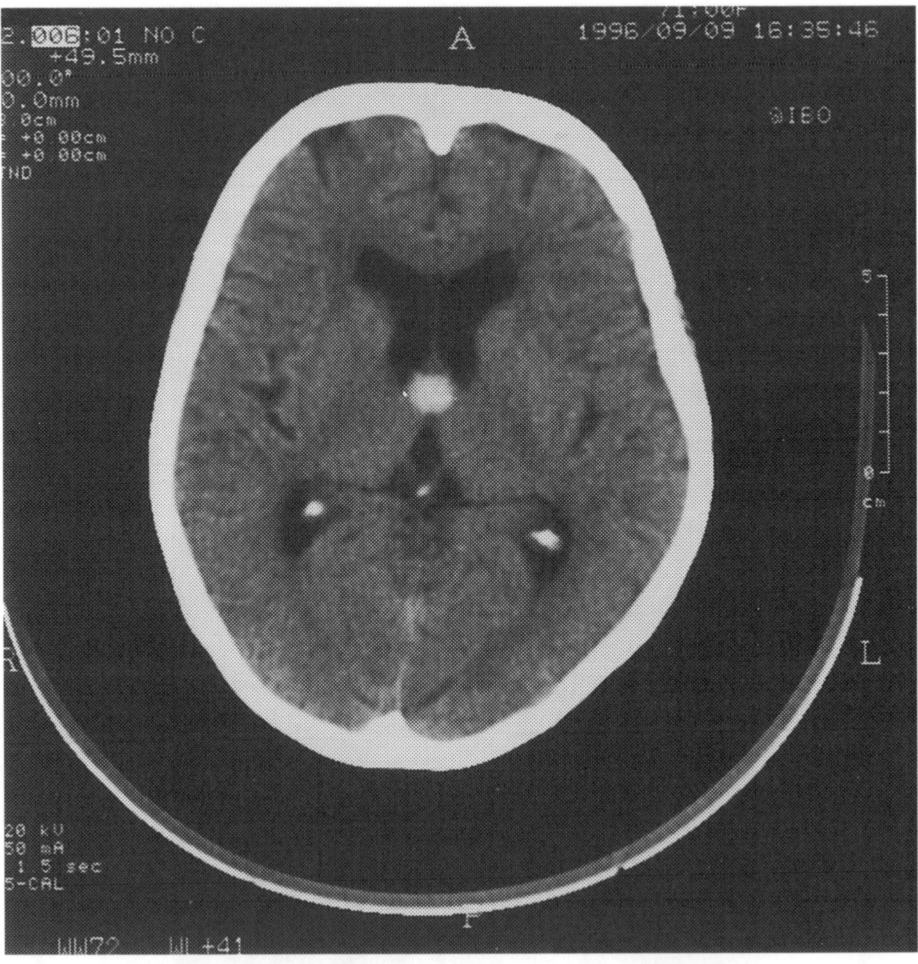

Question 31

This is a retinal photograph of a young man with a mild spastic paraparesis.

(a) Describe the appearance.
(b) What is the probable diagnosis?

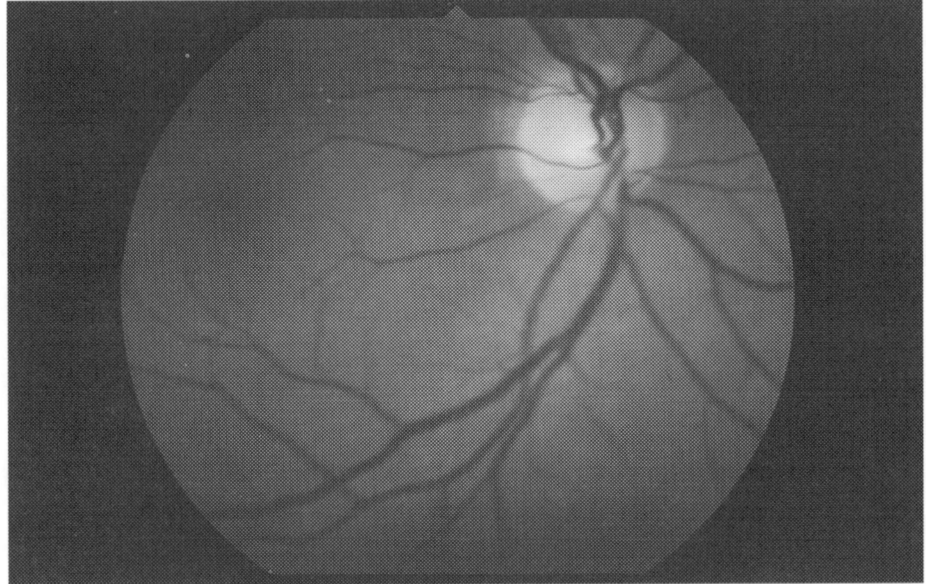

See Slide 6, Colour Plate Section

Question 32

What is the cause of this woman's progressive gait disturbance?

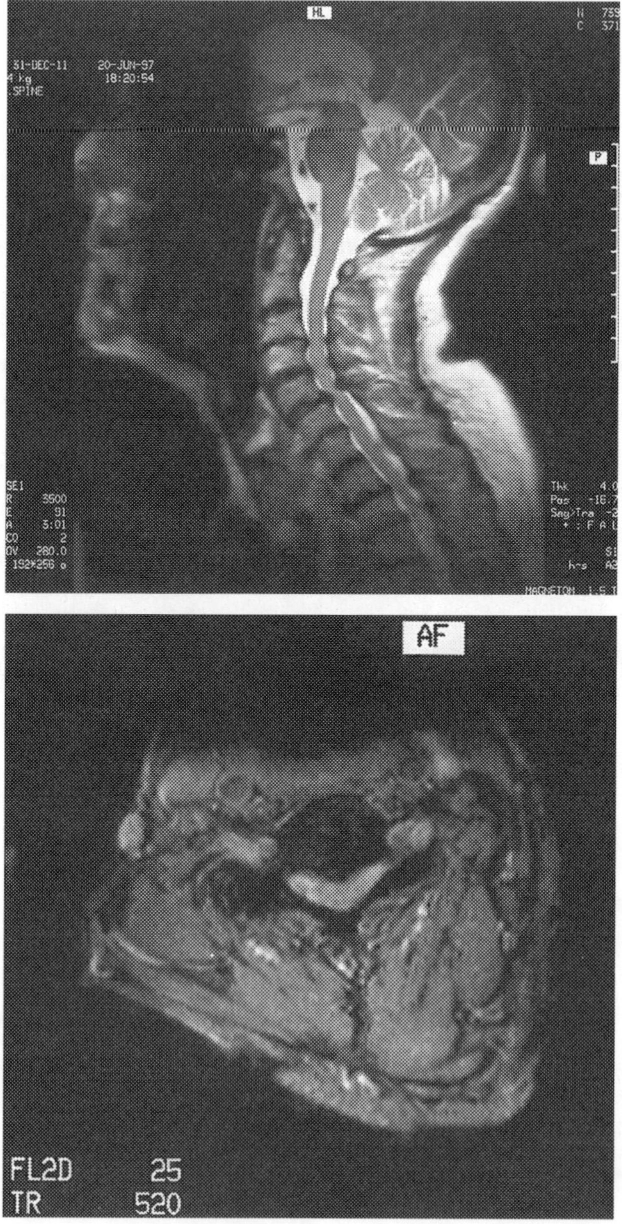

Question 33

After stopping cycling on a regular basis, this man noticed that his jeans were less tight on the left thigh. Examination revealed thinning of the leg, brisk reflexes and extensor plantar responses.

(a) What is the radiological sign?
(b) Explain the neurological presentation.

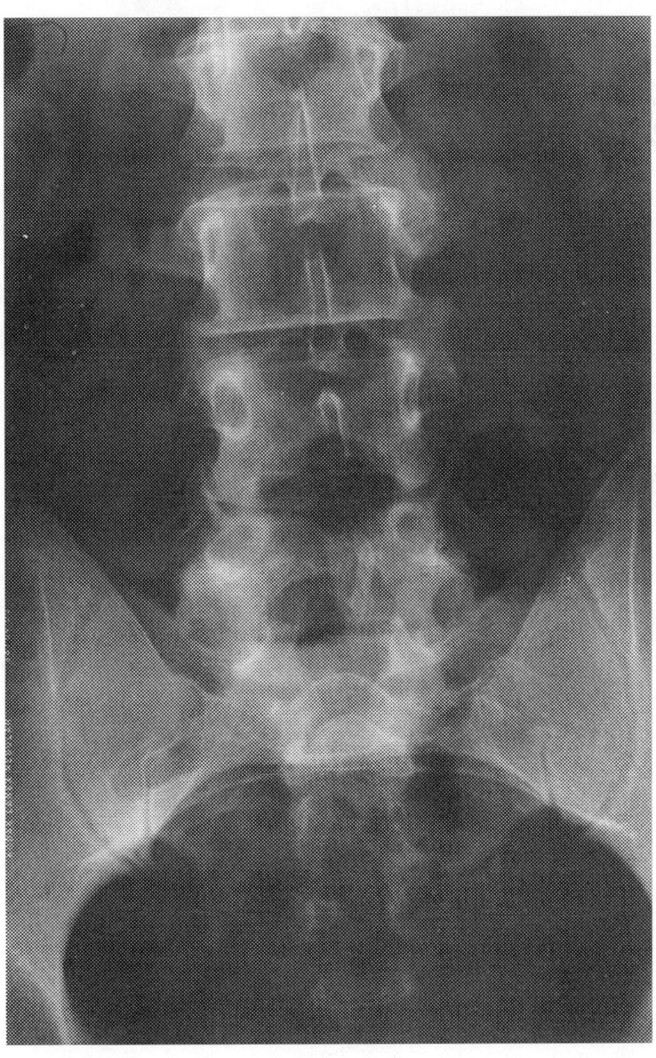

Question 34

(a) What physical signs are evident?
(b) Name two possible sites of the lesion, stating which is more likely.
(c) What treatment can affect prognosis?

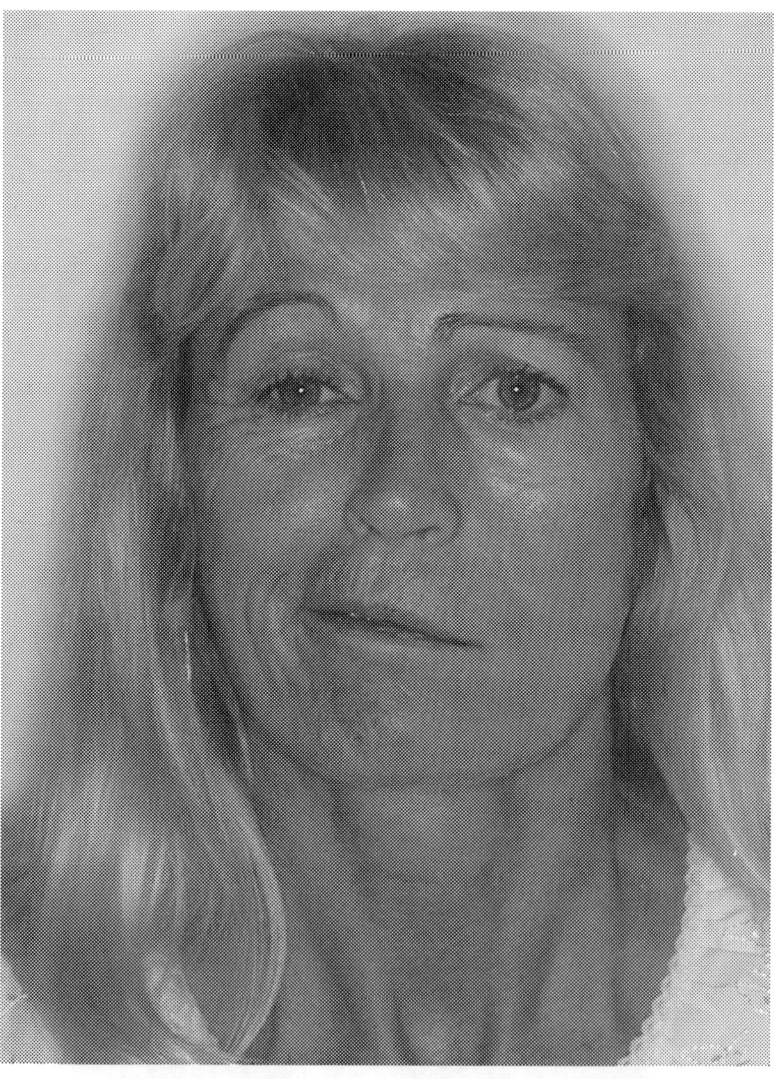

Question 35

This woman presented with a 4-year history of progressive clumsiness/weakness of her right-sided limbs.

(a) What is the underlying pathology?
(b) What is the prognosis?

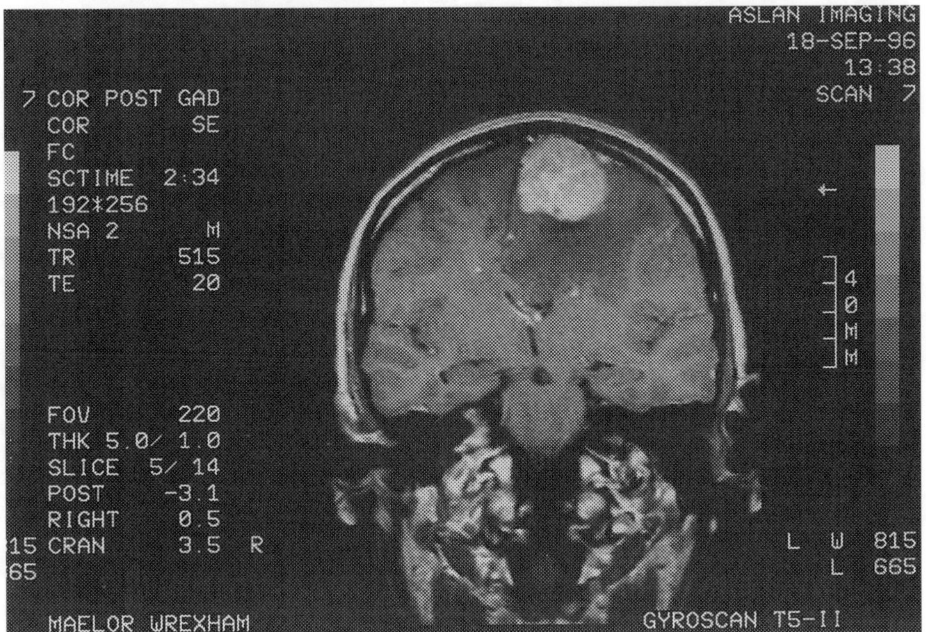

Question 36

(a) Describe these radiological appearances.
(b) What is the likeliest pathology?

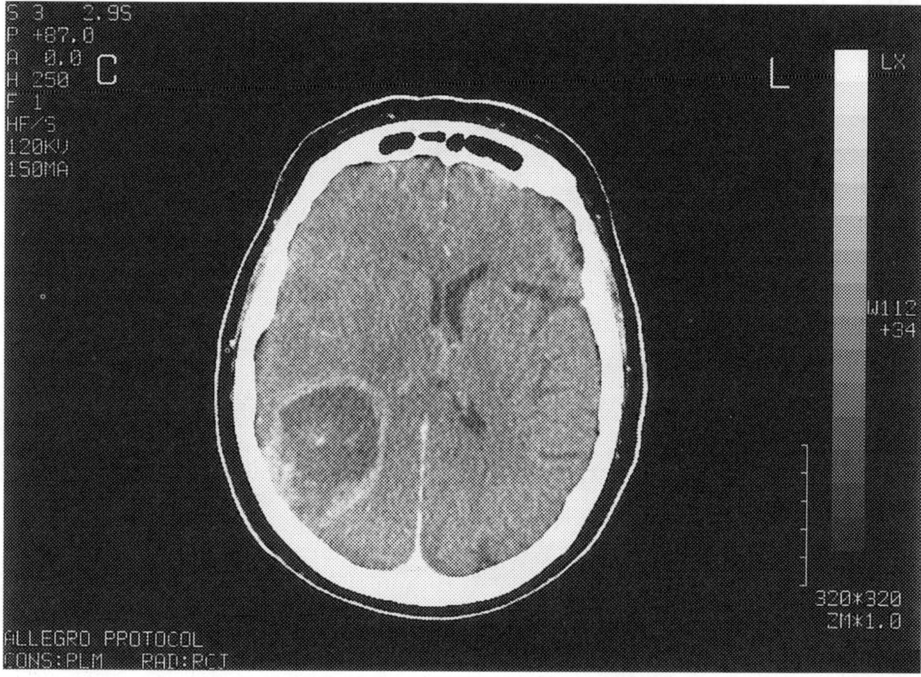

Question 37

This young woman complains of headache and intermittent blurring of vision. CT and MRI scans are normal.

(a) What does the retinal photograph reveal?
(b) What is the diagnosis?
(c) What is the prognosis?

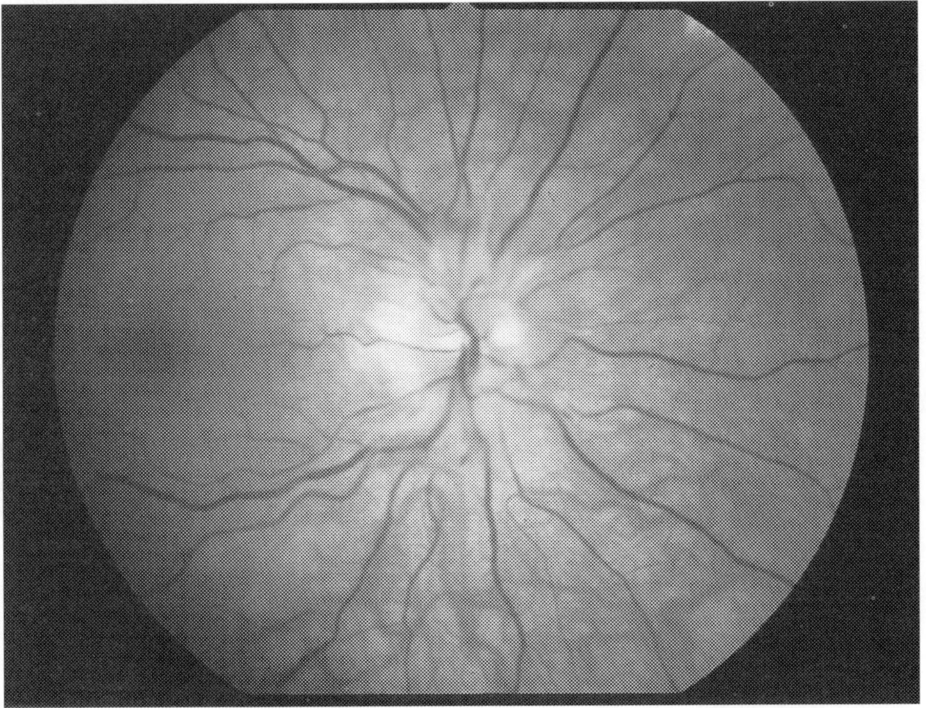

See Slide 7, Colour Plate Section

Question 38

(a) Name this clinical sign.
(b) What is the commonest cause?

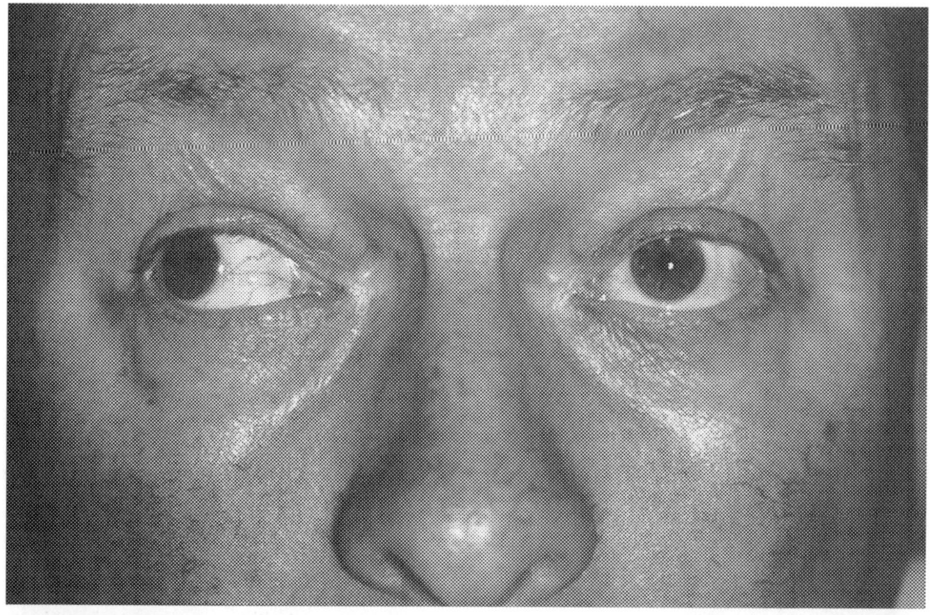

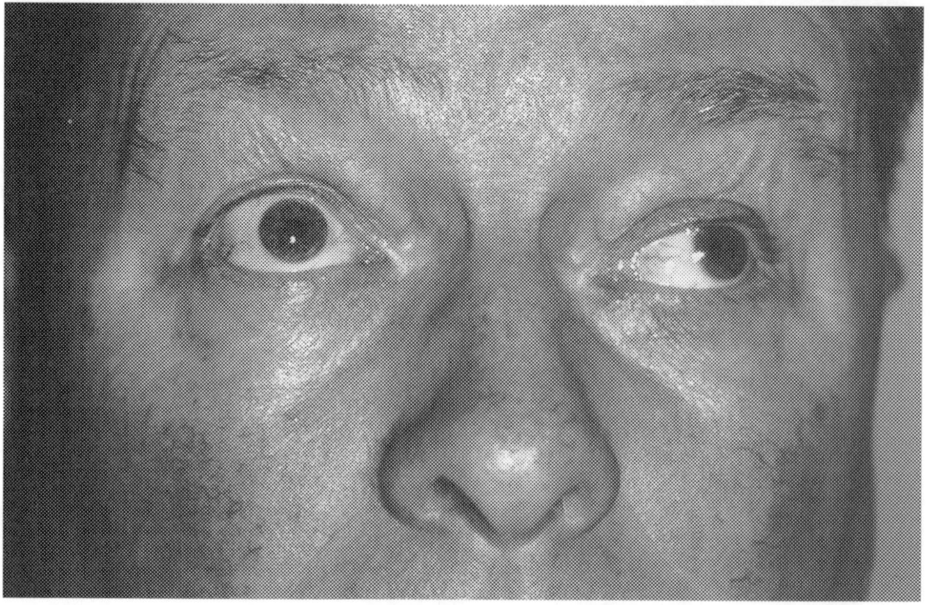

Question 39

A cerebral biopsy was performed on a patient with rapidly deteriorating consciousness and fever but non-specific findings on CT, EEG and CSF.

(a) What is the diagnosis?
(b) Which non-invasive technique permits accurate diagnosis of this condition?

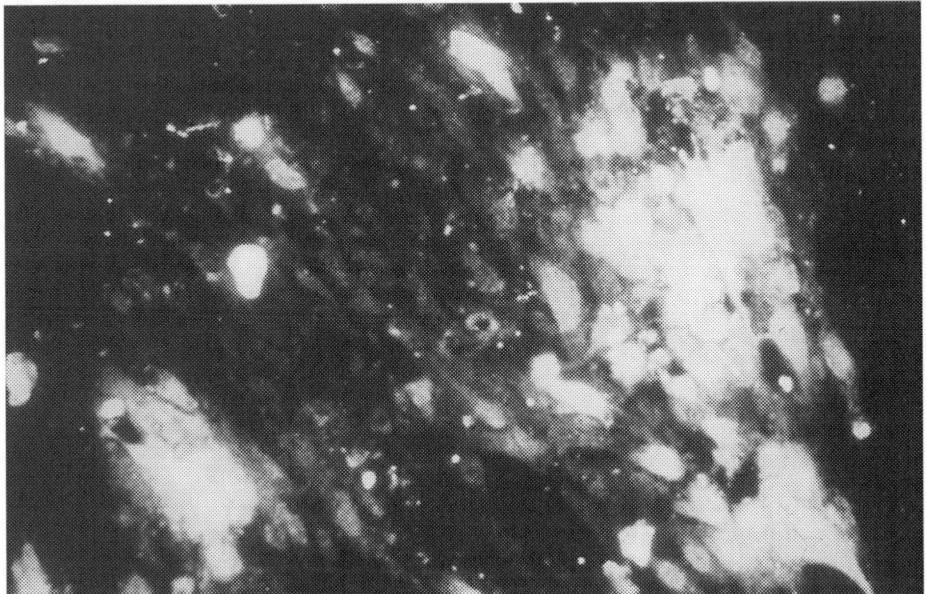

See Slide 8, Colour Plate Section

Question 40

(a) Name this lesion.
(b) What is its clinical significance (prognosis)?

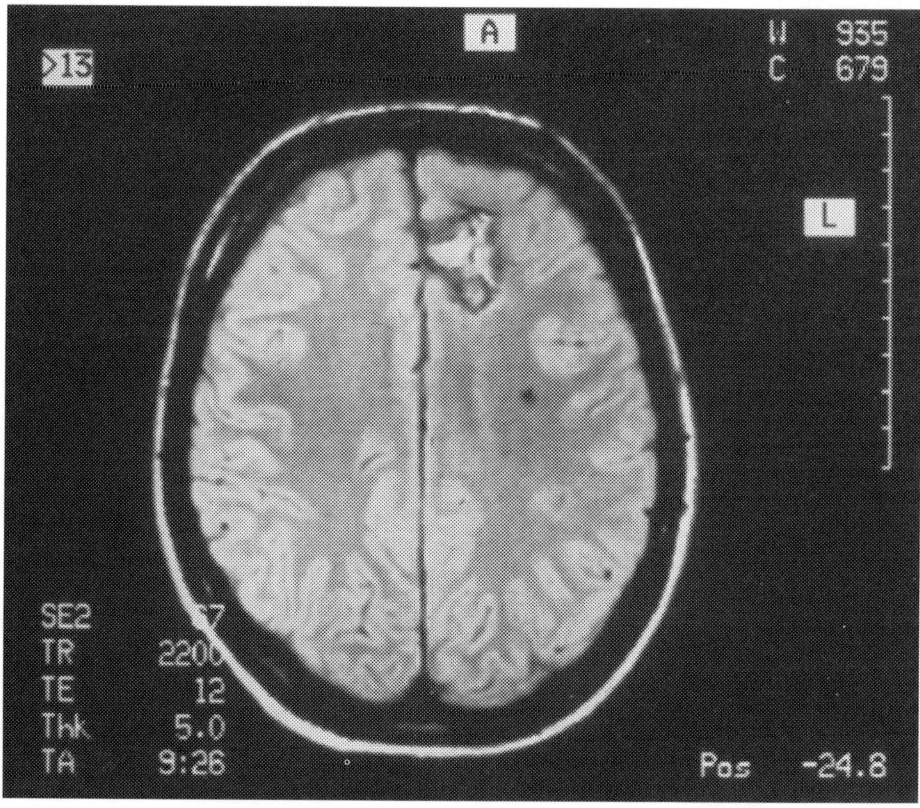

Answer 1

(a) Adenoma sebaceum is the commonest cutaneous manifestation of tuberous sclerosis (TS).
(b) TS is inherited as an autosomal dominant trait with incomplete penetrance.

Answer 2

An acute subdural haematoma. There is an extensive hyperdense lesion overlying the surface of the brain which follows the curve of the inner table of the skull.

Answer 3

(a) Railroad track or 'tramline' calcification.
(b) The characteristic venous malformation (leptomeningeal angiomatosis) of the Sturge–Weber syndrome has a propensity for the occipital or occipitoparietal regions.

Answer 4

(a) The 'ragged red fibre' is a non-specific morphological finding which is common to the mitochondrial cytopathies, a heterogenous group of conditions with diverse clinical presentations.
(b) Myoclonic epilepsy with ragged red fibres (MERRF).

Answer 5

(a) Extensive hypointensity in the pons characteristic of central pontine myelinolysis. The clinical picture is one of spastic quadriplegia, pseudobulbar palsy and 'locked-in syndrome'.
(b) Profound hyponatraemia with rapid correction (>12 mmol/l per day) or absolute correction of hyponatraemia by > 25 mmol/l per day. The rate of correction is more important than the absolute sodium concentration.
(c) The 6-month survival is 5–10% and most survivors are usually severely disabled. Rarely, good recovery occurs, the clinical improvement predating resolution of the MR abnormalities.

Answer 6

(a) Wasting of the thenar eminence, specifically abductor pollicis brevis.
(b) Compression of the median nerve at the wrist (carpal tunnel syndrome).

Answer 7

(a) Primary cerebral lymphoma. CT reveals a homogeneously enhancing mass in the right frontal region with extensive surrounding oedema. Patients with long-term immunosuppression, especially after renal transplantation, are at particular risk of developing this malignancy.
(b) Steroids may produce a dramatic clinical and radiological improvement, but the response is temporary and median survival is 24 months.

Answer 8

Central or type 2 neurofibromatosis. The MR scan reveals bilateral acoustic neuromas and a left sphenoidal wing meningioma. Intrinsic cerebral and optic nerve gliomas are also seen in this condition.

Answer 9

Bilateral caudate atrophy is typical of Huntington's disease. The bulge in the inferolateral border of the lateral ventricle, normally created by the head of the caudate nucleus, has been obliterated.

Answer 10

Chronic progressive external ophthalmoplegia, one of the mitochondrial cytopathies, is the likeliest cause of bilateral ptosis and complete ophthalmoplegia. Myasthenia gravis rarely produces these appearances.

Answer 11

The X-ray reveals a neuropathic knee joint. Analgesic joints, when repeatedly traumatized, may disintegrate. These appearances are classically associated with tabes dorsalis and hereditary sensory neuropathies. These conditions are rare and, today, diabetic sensory neuropathy is the commonest cause.

Answer 12

This man presented with sudden onset of weakness affecting the left arm and face. The CT scan shows a large infarct in the territory of the right middle cerebral artery.

Answer 13

Left Horner's syndrome; ptosis and miosis (small pupil).

Answer 14

A high left internal carotid artery dissection. The scan reveals an eccentrically placed high signal lesion within the wall of the proximal left internal carotid artery. For comparison, one can see a normal flow void within the right internal carotid artery. This commonly presents with a painful Horner's syndrome. Prior to the advent of MRI/MRA this presentation often went unexplained.

Answer 15

Chronic anticonvulsant therapy. Gingival hypertrophy occurs in one third of patients receiving long-term phenytoin. It is less commonly seen with phenobarbitone.

Answer 16

(a) Depressed fracture in the left parietal region. The fracture is comminuted and large fragments are depressed into the brain.
(b) These injuries, which may not produce loss of consciousness, are associated with a 25% risk of post-traumatic epilepsy.

Answer 17

Right third nerve palsy. Her right eyelid is being forcibly elevated (ptosis), there is failure of adduction of the right eye (medial rectus palsy) and the pupil is dilated. Pupillary involvement is more likely with extrinsic compression of the third cranial nerve.

Answer 18

(a) The MR venogram reveals that the cortical veins are running down from, rather than up towards, the sagittal sinus, which is not patent.
(b) Sagittal sinus thrombosis. The puerperal period is associated with an increased risk of venous sinus thrombosis.
(c) Intravenous heparin. While cerebral imaging often reveals the presence of haemorrhages, these are secondary to venous infarction and, therefore, anticoagulation is probably indicated.

Answer 19

The MRI reveals a tumour, arising from the pituitary region, extending superiorly to compress the optic chiasm and impinging upon the left cavernous sinus, visible as displacement of the left carotid artery.

Pituitary tumours may be sub-divided according to size. Lesions less than 1 cm (microadenomas) present with endocrine problems (amenorrhoea-galactorrhoea (prolactin), acromegaly (growth hormone), Cushings Disease (ACTH), hypopituitarism). Lesions greater than 1 cm (macroadenomas) present in a similar manner but as the lesion expands beyond the sella turcica compression effects occur. Most commonly chiasmal compression produces complete or partial bitemporal hemianopia but a variety of other field defects are well-recognised. In 5–10% of cases the lesion causes a cavernous sinus syndrome whose full extent involves ophthalmoplegia with loss of sensation in the ophthalmic division of the trigeminal nerve. Rarer presentations, caused by invasion of adjacent structures, include seizures (temporal lobe), CSF rhinorrhoea (cribriform plate), diabetes insipidus (posterior pituitary), hypothermia and somnolence (hypothalamus).

Answer 20

(a) Moya Moya disease. The angiogram reveals the classical 'puff of smoke' sign caused by an anastomotic network of perforating arteries consequent upon occlusion of the terminal portions of both internal carotid arteries. A normal right carotid angiogram (right) is shown for comparison. While first described in Japanese children, the condition is now well-recognized in the West. It has been described as a consequence of radiotherapy to the pituitary fossa and chronic basal meningitides, but most cases are idiopathic.
(b) The commonest presentations are TIAs/stroke in childhood, and sub-arachnoid haemorrage in juveniles and young adults.

Answer 21

Alzheimer's disease. This specimen reveals neurofibrillary tangles in virtually every large neurone and neuritic plaques are also seen.

Answer 22

(a) Numerous small areas of calcification throughout both hemispheres highly suggestive of neurocysticercosis.
(b) Epilepsy. This is the commonest cause of epilepsy in some parts of the developing world. Early treatment with praziquantel abolishes the need for anticonvulsant therapy in 70% of cases but if lesions calcify a permanent epileptic focus may result.
(c) Other cerebral manifestations include focal deficits, obstructive hydrocephalus and subarachnoid haemorrhage.

Answer 23

(a) Left scapular winging due to weakness of serratus anterior.
(b) Traumatic damage to the left long thoracic nerve.

Answer 24

(a) Multiple periventricular high-intensity lesions.
(b) While multiple sclerosis is the commonest cause, cerebral lupus can produce indistinguishable appearances. Diagnosis, therefore, depends mainly on clinical and other investigative findings.

Answer 25

(a) A left posterior communicating artery aneurysm.
(b) While classically associated with painful third nerve palsy, the commonest presentation is a subarachnoid haemorrhage.

Answer 26

(a) Toxoplasma abscess. Extensive low-density change in the left hemisphere within which lies an enhancing area with a slightly denser rim.
(b) Empirical treatment with sulfadiazine and pyrimethamine. If no

improvement occurs within 2 weeks, brain biopsy is required to exclude other causes. Since this represents reactivation of a pre-existing infection, lifelong treatment is required.

Answer 27

(a) Heliotrope discoloration of the cheeks best seen infraorbitally and peri-orbital/eyelid oedema. These are characteristic features of dermatomyositis.
(b) Painless proximal muscle weakness (polymyositis).
(c) Twenty per cent of patients make a full recovery and a further 20% achieve prolonged remissions with steroid therapy. Adverse prognostic factors include delayed treatment and coexistent malignancy, present in up to 50% of patients with dermatomyositis/polymyositis with onset in middle age.

Answer 28

(a) Severe atrophy of the brainstem, particularly the pons, and the cerebellum. The clinical picture and scan appearances suggest olivopontocerebellar atrophy.
(b) This is one of the conditions which may bear a superficial resemblance to idiopathic Parkinson's disease but should be distinguished by the other clinical features, the relentlessly progressive course and the lack of response to dopamine replacement therapy.

Answer 29

(a) Total blockage of the downward passage of radiographic contrast medium.
(b) An obstructive process, probably malignant, within the spinal sub-arachnoid space. Infective (tuberculosis) and granulomatous conditions (sarcoidosis) are less common causes of this appearance.

Answer 30

(a) Colloid cyst of the third ventricle. There is a small, round, uniformly enhancing lesion situated in the anterior portion of the ventricle and attached to the roof of the ventricle.
(b) Intermittent severe bifrontal/bioccipital headaches due to 'ball-valve' obstruction of the third ventricle. Sudden crises of headache, obtundation,

unsteadiness, incontinence, weakness and drop attacks without loss of consciousness.

Answer 31

(a) Pallor of the optic disc with a well-defined margin and normal retinal vasculature.
(b) Multiple sclerosis. Given his other clinical findings, the retinal photograph probably represents previous optic neuritis.

Answer 32

Cervical spondylitic myelopathy. The sagittal images reveal extensive degenerative changes. Cord compression (confirmed on the axial image) is caused by a combination of anterior osteophytosis and posterior ligamentous hypertrophy.

Answer 33

(a) Spina bifida (L5 level).
(b) Failure of vertebral fusion is associated with tethering of the nerve roots in the cauda equina. As the individual grows the nerve roots and the terminal portion of the spinal cord become stretched and damaged. Hence the combination of upper and lower motor neurone signs.

Answer 34

(a) Drooping of the corner of the mouth, effacement of skin creases, widening of the palpebral fissure and failure to elevate the left eyebrow.
(b) This is a lower motor neurone-type left seventh nerve palsy. Complete facial weakness can be seen in nuclear lesions but a peripheral lesion (Bell's palsy) is most likely.
(c) High-dose prednisolone, given within a few days of onset, may be beneficial.

Answer 35

(a) Left parietal meningioma. MR reveals characteristic appearance of a uniformly enhancing lesion arising from the meninges. This is compressing the underlying brain producing extensive oedema.

(b) Excision of the lesion should prevent further deterioration. While improvement often occurs, complete recovery of function is unusual. There is a significant risk of epilepsy and 10–15% of meningiomas recur or undergo malignant transformation.

Answer 36

(a) There is an irregular mass in the right parieto-occipital region with mass effect (obliteration of the lateral ventricle and right-to-left shift). The wall shows enhancement but the centre is of low density suggesting necrosis or cystic change.
(b) Malignant glioma. The CT appearance suggests a very aggressive lesion, possibly a glioblastoma multiforme.

Answer 37

(a) Papilloedema.
(b) Benign intracranial hypertension.
(c) This is not a life-threatening condition but the description 'benign' can be misleading. In most cases, medical therapy, weight reduction, diuretics, repeated lumbar punctures or steroids are effective. However, chronically raised intracranial pressure presents a serious threat to vision. Visual obscurations are an ominous symptom and visual failure can occur suddenly. Where medical treatment is unsuccessful, surgery, optic nerve fenestration or ventriculo-peritoneal shunting is necessary.

Answer 38

(a) Bilateral internuclear ophthalmoplegia (INO). There is failure of adduction of the left (top picture) and right eyes (bottom picture). This will usually be accompanied by nystagmus of the abducting eye. This is caused by lesions of the medial longitudinal fasiculus which connects the third nerve nucleus with the contralateral sixth nerve nucleus.
(b) Multiple sclerosis. Unilateral INO may be caused by vascular events, tumours or granulomata, but demyelination is by far the commonest cause of bilateral INO.

Answer 39

(a) *Herpes simplex* encephalitis. Immunofluorescence of the temporal lobe reveals the presence of fluorescent-labelled antibody and, therefore, abundant *Herpes simplex* antigen.

(b) Polymerase chain reaction. Amplification of *Herpes simplex* virus (HSV)-specific DNA in the CSF can confirm/refute this diagnosis within 24 hours. Even prior to the advent of this technique, brain biopsy was mainly indicated to exclude other pathologies. If *Herpes simplex* encephalitis is considered, intravenous acyclovir should be commenced without delay.

Answer 40

(a) Cavernous angioma. A partly serpiginous lesion in the left medial frontal region. A surrounding dark 'halo', caused by haemosiderin, is characteristic.
(b) These lesions cause drug-resistant epilepsy and represent up to 5% of cases seen in large surgical series. While the MR appearances are characteristic, CT scans are often unremarkable. The epilepsy is probably the consequence of repeated leakages into surrounding tissue. Unlike arteriovenous malformations, these lesions rarely produce massive haemorrhage.

Viva Topics

Viva 1

Discuss the management of acute Guillain–Barré syndrome

In the management of any condition, one must: (1) establish the diagnosis; (2) assess severity; (3) treat the underlying condition (if applicable); and institute (4) general supportive measures and (5) specific therapies.

1. Acute Guillain–Barré syndrome presents with progressive limb weakness, usually over a few days, often following recovery from an infective illness. Examination reveals limb weakness varying from mild distal weakness to quadriplegia, with flaccidity and areflexia and, usually, no hard sensory signs. Involvement of facial, respiratory and bulbar muscles is not uncommon.

   Diagnosis is confirmed by nerve conduction studies which reveal a patchy demyelinating motor neuropathy (grossly delayed motor nerve conduction velocities, conduction block, normal sensory action potentials). These 'classical features' may not be present if the neurophysiology is carried out too early but treatment should not be delayed if the clinical picture is suggestive. Other variants are pure axonal, mixed axonal and demyelinating, and, with prominent sensory abnormalities, are well described. The CSF protein is usually markedly elevated and there should be no cells.

2. The mortality rate varies from 1.5% to 15% with the lowest rates reported by specialist centres. Adverse prognostic factors include increasing age, explosive onset, the axonal variant, following *Campylobacter* enteritis and the need for ventilatory support. Approximately 20% of patients have a permanent neurological deficit. While 70% 'recover fully', it is not yet known what proportion return to their previous level of activity.

4. General supportive measures have a significant influence both in saving life and preventing complications. Vital issues include airway security and prevention of aspiration, prompt treatment of chest infections, continuous ECG/blood pressure monitoring and treatment of autonomic instability, particularly cardiac dysrhythmia, early recognition and treatment of paralytic ileus, prophylaxis against thromboembolism, maintenance of adequate nutrition, effective management of pain, passive physiotherapy to prevent limb contractures, and communication aids in patients who are bed-bound with a tracheostomy *in situ*.

5. Controlled clinical trials have shown that corticosteroids are of no benefit. In the mid-1980s, plasma exchange, presumably by removal of an unidentified myelotoxic agent, was proven to 'speed up recovery', resulting in shorter time on ventilation, in intensive care unit (ICU) and in hospital.

However, this treatment had no influence on the proportion of severely disabled patients at 1-year follow-up. In 1992, intravenous immunoglobulin was shown to be as efficacious as plasma exchange. Whilst there were suggestions that this trial was biased in favour of intravenous immunoglobulin, subsequent evidence supports its main conclusion.

The ongoing Plasma Exchange Sandoglobulin Guillain–Barré Study (PSGBS) is a three-armed, controlled clinical trial comparing intravenous immunoglobulin, plasma exchange or both treatments. Preliminary data suggest no difference in the early outcome. Unless there are differences in percentage severe disability, the choice of treatment will probably depend on other factors. In this regard, whilst intravenous immunoglobulin is expensive, this form of treatment is readily available, simple and associated with few problems: allergy, aseptic meningitis, migraine, stroke and renal failure are all rare complications. Transmission of HIV or hepatitis B surface antigen (HbSAg) has not been described.

References

Guillain–Barré Syndrome Study Group. Plasmapheresis and acute Guillain–Barré syndrome. *Neurology* 1984, **35**, 1096–104.

van der Meche FGA, Schimtz PIM and the Dutch Guillain–Barré Study Group. A randomised trial comparing intravenous immune globulin and plasma exchange in Guillain–Barré. *N Engl J Med* 1992, **326**, 1123–9.

Viva 2

Narcoleptic syndrome

This has been defined as a disorder of unknown aetiology, which is characterized by excessive sleepiness that typically is associated with cataplexy and other REM sleep phenomena, such as sleep paralysis and hypnagogic hallucinations.

Reported prevalence rates vary but are probably approximately $50/10^5$, i.e. 30000 cases in the UK. Under-reporting is likely as the condition often remains unrecognized for many years. Patients most commonly present between the ages of 15 and 25.

The diagnosis can usually be achieved on clinical grounds only: in the presence of excessive daytime sleepiness, the recognition of cataplexy is the key factor. Cataplexy may be defined as laughter-induced, loss of facial and jaw control spreading to involve the trunk and other bodily areas, accompanied by muscle jerking around the mouth. It often culminates in a fall and injuries are common. Sleep paralysis is the inability to move during the transition between sleep and wakefulness and is associated with a feeling of terror. This occurs more commonly in the narcoleptic syndrome than other sleep–wake disorders but is not the diagnostic equivalent of cataplexy. True hypnagogic hallucinations are not a feature of this condition. The actual complaint is the frequent occurrence of vivid dreams at sleep onset. Additional clinical features include disturbed sleep (short sleep latency, frequent arousal, reduced total sleep time) and motor dyscontrol (muscle jerks, sleep walking and sleep talking).

In clear-cut cases, laboratory investigation is for research purposes only. However, in the absence of cataplexy, confident clinical diagnosis may be impossible. Metabolic causes of hypersomnolence, idiopathic hypersomnia and obstructive sleep apnoea should be considered. In these patients, complete laboratory investigations may be useful: the multiple sleep latency test usually reveals mean sleep onset latency of less than 7 minutes. Polysomnography can demonstrate frequent awakening and fragmented REM periods. While there is no specific genetic marker, 90% of patients possess HLA-DR2 compared to 20–30% of unaffected individuals.

The narcolepsy syndrome is a lifelong condition which rarely remits, causes significant physical and psychosocial disability and traditional treatment is unsatisfactory. While excessive daytime somnolence is often treated with centrally acting stimulants, there have been no large-scale controlled trials of their efficacy and tolerability. These drugs possess limited efficacy, cause prominent sympathomimetic adverse effects, carry significant risk of rebound hypersomnolence and are subject to tolerance. Cataplexy usually responds to serotonin reuptake inhibitors (clomipramine, fluoxetine). Combination therapies are hampered by adverse effects: sweating, increased appetite, weight gain and impaired sexual function.

A promising, novel, wake-promoting agent, modafinil, has recently received a product licence in the UK. Preclinical evaluation demonstrates that it increases wake time and consolidates wakefulness without the risk of rebound hypersomnolence, psychomotor stimulation or anxiety. Its lack of dopaminergic activity means that euphoria does not occur and that it has a low potential for abuse in humans. In one large randomized controlled trial comparing two doses of modafinil with a placebo, the active compound was effective in maintaining wakefulness and was well tolerated, producing only headaches and dry mouth significantly more frequently than the placebo.

References

Parkes JD, Clift SJ, Dahlitz MJ, Chen SY, Dunn G. The narcoleptic syndrome. *J Neurol Neurosurg Psychiat* 1995, **59**, 221–4.

Viva 3

Describe the management of generalized convulsive status epilepticus in an adult in the hospital setting

Generalized convulsive status epilepticus (GCSE) can be defined as either two or more convulsive seizures without an intervening period of full recovery of consciousness, or as recurrent epileptic seizures lasting for more than 30 minutes. GCSE is a common medical emergency with a diverse aetiology which is the principal determinant of outcome. The next most important predictor of outcome is the duration of status and, therefore, delays in the institution of effective therapy may contribute to an adverse outcome in some cases.

Making the diagnosis

Diagnosis requires questioning witnesses about the duration of the attack and any treatment already given. Relatives or acquaintances should be asked if there is any history of seizures, alcohol or drug abuse, metabolic or vascular disease, head trauma or recent neurological symptoms. If the patient is known to have epilepsy, an attempt should be made to discover whether the seizures or treatment have recently changed. This brief history will help to determine treatment and the need for investigations.

Overt GCSE must be differentiated from pseudostatus. Admitting doctors should be suspicious of the 'known epileptic', with a history of repeated 'status epilepticus' despite polytherapy, who presents with fluctuating, often semi-purposeful limb movements. Findings on examination include resistance to passive eye-opening, persistence of positive conjunctival reflex, downgoing plantar responses and apparently repeated generalized seizures without cyanosis. These patients are often admitted to intensive care unit after iatrogenic respiratory arrest because they have been exposed to multiple doses of intravenous benzodiazepines with or without chlormethiazole infusions. Correct management involves observation and reassurance of patient, relatives and staff.

Treatment

The aims of treatment are the rapid control of seizures, prevention of systemic complications and treatment of the underlying cause. Management takes place in phases which reflect the underlying pathophysiology. While a timed sequence is described, the process is continuous. For simplicity, the specific and general measures are combined.

Early status (0–30 minutes)

A single bolus of a rapidly acting benzodiazepine, 10 mg diazepam or 4 mg lorazepam, will abolish seizures in 70–80% of cases. A second bolus is required if seizures persist or recur after 20–30 minutes. Respiratory depression or hypotension occurs in up to 13% of patients receiving either benzodiazepine.

Whichever drug is given, blood glucose should be checked at the bedside to exclude hypoglycaemia. If the patient is hypoglycaemic, 50 ml 50% dextrose should be given intravenously. If the patient is thought to chronically abuse alcohol, 250 mg thiamine should be administered by slow intravenous injection (over 10 minutes) and facilities for treating anaphylactic shock should be available.

Heart rate, blood pressure, ECG, temperature and neurological status should be assessed regularly. An intravenous line should be established and physiological saline infused to keep it patent. It is best to use a large vein to minimize the risk of phlebitis when antiepileptic drugs are given. Blood should be taken for the measurement of blood glucose, urea, electrolytes (including calcium and magnesium), acid–base balance, liver function, full blood count, clotting, antiepileptic drug and alcohol concentrations. Blood should be cultured if the patient is febrile. Spare samples should be stored so that further tests can be carried out later if required.

If the patient has recently stopped taking an antiepileptic drug, this should be restarted as soon as possible. The patient should be examined for evidence of head trauma, meningeal irritation, focal neurological deficit, an underlying metabolic condition or drug abuse, and treated accordingly. Whether the patient will require more specific investigations such as cerebral imaging or cerebrospinal fluid examination will depend on the initial assessment and response to treatment.

Established status epilepticus (30–90 minutes)

GCSE is considered established if it continues for 30 minutes despite initial therapy. The patient should be transferred to an intensive care unit and treated with either intravenous phenytoin or phenobarbitone. If facilities are available, management should also include continuous or frequent monitoring of intra-arterial pressure, central venous pressure, blood gases and pulmonary wedge pressure. The recommended loading dose of phenytoin is 15 mg/kg, with further boluses up to 30 mg/kg if seizures persist. The infusion rate should not exceed 50 mg/minute, to minimize the risk of cardiac dysrhythmias, and phenytoin should not be injected via the same giving set as diazepam because of the possibility of crystallization. The dose of phenobarbitone is 15 mg/kg at a rate of no greater than 100 mg/minute. This drug can cause hypotension, sedation and respiratory depression, but these effects usually only occur with high doses.

Refractory status epilepticus (60–90 minutes)

If GCSE persists despite the above measures, it is considered refractory. Pseudostatus should be considered and adherence to the treatment protocol checked. The next step is to give a general anaesthetic, provide ventilation, haemodynamic and organ support, and treatment of the underlying cause, e.g. meningitis. Traditionally, intravenous thiopentone has been the drug of first choice. It is given in a dose of 75–125 mg over 10–15 seconds and repeated if necessary. Hypotension requiring inotropic support is a common complication. This drug has a long elimination half-life and accumulates during prolonged infusion, thus delaying recovery after cessation of treatment. Recently intravenous propofol has been used increasingly in intensive care units in the UK. While it has the advantage of rapid onset and recovery, it can cause bradycardia and there are reports of pro-convulsant activity. More information is required before it can be recommended for routine use.

References

Stopping status epilepticus. *Drugs Therapeut Bull* 1996, **34**, 73–6.

Viva 4

Discuss the role of interferon-beta in the management of patients with multiple sclerosis

Multiple sclerosis affects approximately 80 000 people in the UK. Three clinical courses are recognized. In the majority (80%), the illness is characterized by relapses and remissions, but, ultimately, progressive disability. In 5%, the condition is progressive from the onset, while the remaining 15% follow a 'benign' course with full recovery of relapses and little or no accumulating functional deficit.

The aetiology is not fully understood, but it is widely accepted that a combination of genetic, environmental and autoimmune factors is involved. In the last two decades, the search for treatments has focused on compounds with immunoregulatory effects. However, the development of effective disease-modifying agents is hampered by a lack of understanding of aetiology/pathophysiology and by the complex relationship between the acute clinical presentations, the MR findings and the development of disability.

Interferon beta 1b

A total of 372 patients with relapsing/remitting MS were randomized to receive placebo, low-dose (1.6 MIU) or high-dose (8 MIU) interferon beta 1b by subcutaneous injection on an alternate day basis. All patients were aged between 18 and 50 years, had experienced at least two relapses in the previous 2 years and were able to walk at least 100 metres unaided without resting. When first published, 286 patients had been followed-up for 2 years while the final publication included 164 patients.

At 2 years, the relapse rate was significantly lower in the high-dose treatment group (0.8/patient/year) than in those receiving placebo (1.27/patient/year). Thirty-six patients in the high-dose group remained relapse-free compared to 18 in the placebo group. The secondary end points were based on MR appearances. At 2 years, the total area of abnormality had increased by 20% in the placebo group and was unchanged in the high-dose treatment group. Neutralizing antibodies developed in 45% of those in the high-dose treatment group and this correlated with an increase in relapse rate at 18–24 months.

Eighty-two per cent in the high-dose group developed flu-like symptoms at the onset of treatment which were usually controlled with non-steroidal anti-inflammatory drugs (NSAIDs). Skin irritation at the injection site occurred in 80%, falling to 50% with the passage of time, and could be reduced by taking antihistamines or varying the injection site. Depression occurred twice as commonly in the high-dose group than in the placebo group.

The results of this study must be interpreted with caution. The analysis used was not intention to treat, which may have introduced a bias in favour of the active compound. Furthermore, 20% of relapses were not medically verified and, when these are excluded, there was no difference in the number of exacerbation-free patients between the placebo and high-dose treatment groups. Finally, while there was a trend towards lesser disability, as measured by the Kurtzke extended disability status scale (EDSS), in high-dose relative to placebo, this did not reach statistical significance.

Interferon beta 1a

A total of 301 patients with mild to moderate relapsing/remitting MS aged betwen 18 and 55 years were randomized to receive placebo ($n = 143$) or 6 MIU interferon beta 1a ($n = 158$) by weekly intramuscular injections. The primary outcome variable was time to sustained progression, defined as deterioration from baseline by at least 1 point on the EDSS persisting for at least 6 months. All EDSS assessments were conducted by independent physicians. The other clinical outcome measure was time to first exacerbation, all of which were medically verified.

In those completing 2 years (placebo, 87; beta 1a, 85), the annual relapse rate was significantly lower in the treatment group (0.62) than in the placebo group (0.90). Furthermore, the number of exacerbations per patient was significantly higher in those receiving placebo with more than twice as many patients experiencing three or more relapses. More impressively, within the whole group, the primary end point, time to sustained progression of disability, was significantly delayed in the treatment group ($p = 0.024$).

Adverse effects, which were more commonly reported by beta 1a recipients, included flu-like symptoms, muscle aches, asthenia, chills and fever, but skin reactions, depressive symptoms and menstrual irregularity occurred equally frequently in both groups. A total of 22% of interferon beta 1a recipients developed neutralizing antibodies by 104 weeks.

The authors concluded that systematically administered interferon beta 1a significantly slows the progression of sustained neurological disability and is well tolerated in patients with relapsing MS. Furthermore, 'it reduces the frequency of exacerbations and disease activity as measured by serial gadolinium-enhanced MRI' and 'alters the fundamental course of relapsing MS'.

In response, the Association of British Neurologists (ABN) council expressed concern that the study had stopped recruiting before all patients had completed 2 years on the grounds that the total number of patient-years had been reached earlier than anticipated because of an unexpectedly low drop-out rate. It was conceded that, while Kaplan–Meier estimates of the probability of sustained progression were reduced from 34.9% of placebo recipients to 21.9% of interferon recipients, the early termination of the study meant that the actual figures for progression at 2 years were 18/85 versus 29/87, which did not reach statistical significance ($p = 0.07$). Furthermore, patients recruited were at the lower end of the Kurtzke scale, where the influence of impairment is much greater than of disability. Therefore, there was a suggestion of an effect on disability but this could not be regarded as established.

Conclusions

Both interferon beta 1a and 1b have a modest effect in reducing relapse frequency in relapsing/remitting MS. In addition, interferon beta 1a may have a modest effect in slowing the progression of disease, but more data are required before concluding that this effect is established and that there is a real difference between the two compounds. There are, as yet, no published data on the long-term efficacy of these compounds and, given the incidence of neutralizing antibodies, there are genuine fears that this modest degree of efficacy will be lost with the passage of time. There are no published data on the use of interferons in patients with progressive MS. Both compounds seem to be well-tolerated but beta 1b may be associated with an increased risk of depression.

Interferon beta 1b obtained a UK product licence in 1995 and interferon beta 1a received a similar licence in 1997. At a cost of £10 000 per patient per year with approximately 10 000 eligible patients, the potential annual cost to the National Health Service (NHS) is £100m. Additional 'hidden costs' include the time of MS nurses required to train patients/relatives to administer injections, and frequent visits to hospital to monitor the efficacy and safety of these compounds.

The ABN has issued strict guidelines for the utilization of these drugs. They may only be used for ambulant patients with clinically definite MS who are in the relapsing/remitting phase of the disease and who have had at least two disabling attacks of neurological dysfunction in the previous 2 years, followed by recovery which may or may not have been complete. They can only be prescribed by specific named neurologists and individual health authorities have developed mechanisms for funding this treatment. These issues are particularly important given increasing evidence of misuse of interferons in the USA.

References

IFNB Multiple Sclerosis Study Group. Interferon Beta-1b is effective in relapsing–remitting multiple sclerosis. I. Clinical results of a multicentre, randomised double-blind, placebo-controlled trial. *Neurology* 1993, **43**, 655–61.

The IFNB Multiple Sclerosis Study Group, the University of British Columbia MS/MRI Analysis Group. Interferon beta 1b in the treatment of multiple sclerosis: final outcome of the randomised controlled trial. *Neurology* 1995, **45**, 1277–85.

Interferon beta-1b – hope or hype? *Drugs Therapeut Bull* 1996, **34**, 9–11.

Jacobs LD, Cookfair DL, Rudick RA *et al*. Intramuscular interferon beta-1a for disease progression in relapsing multiple sclerosis. *Ann Neurol* 1996, **39**, 285–94.

Viva 5

Discuss the investigation of a 40 year old woman presenting with an infarct in the left middle cerebral artery territory

A total of 12% of first strokes occur before the age of 45, 50% of these are ischaemic and the aetiology is diverse. Some clinical (headache, papilloedema, seizures, impaired consciousness) and radiological features (haemorrhagic infarct) suggest venous infarction, which, in turn, implies conditions predisposing to venous thrombosis (e.g. thrombophilias). Infarction in multiple territories suggests a cardioembolic source or vasculitis, while multiple events within the same arterial territory implicate the feeding vessel. This viva discusses a systematic approach to an individual with a first event in a single arterial territory. Most authorities advocate a simple set of screening tests followed by specific investigations (table), guided by probability and clinical clues, designed to investigate the presence of embolism (extracranial vessels or heart), disease of the intracranial vessels (vasculitis) or prothrombotic states.

History and examination

The clinician should enquire about risk factors for and examine for evidence of atherosclerosis (past history of ischaemic heart disease, hypertension, diabetes mellitus, smoking, cutaneous stigmata of hyperlipidaemia, cholesterol emboli on fundoscopy), and left internal carotid artery dissection (neck or hemicranial pain, recent history of minor head/neck trauma, ipsilateral Horner's or lower cranial nerve palsies).

A cardiac source may be implicated by a history of recent myocardial infarct (mural thrombus), the presence of atrial fibrillation/murmurs (rheumatic, congenital heart disease) or signs of infective endocarditis (fever, splinter haemorrhages, murmurs, Roth spots, microscopic haematuria).

Other clues which should be actively sought include history of recurrent miscarriages, livedo reticularis (antiphospholipid syndrome), past history of deep venous thrombosis or pulmonary embolism (coagulopathies), family history of thromboses (inherited thrombophilias), skin rashes and arthralgia (vasculitides, SLE).

A history of migraine, with focal features, is potentially relevant, particularly if she is a smoker and takes the oral contraceptive pill. Finally, direct questioning about drug abuse and examination for venepuncture marks is essential.

Investigations

Embolism (extracranial vessels, heart)

Initial investigation should concentrate on the left internal carotid artery because atheromatous stenosis accounts for 30–35% and arterial dissection for a further 10–25% of strokes in this age group.

A non-invasive approach is advocated. Ultrasound scanning will reliably detect moderate to severe stenosis and carotid dissection. The success of this technique is very dependent on the operator and, even in expert hands, there can be difficulty distinguishing between very severe stenosis and complete occlusion. Confirmation of ultrasound results by MRI/MRA is recommended. MRA detects stenosis with a high degree of sensitivity and specificity when compared to intra-arterial angiography, which should be reserved for patients with equivocal non-invasive tests or those who cannot tolerate

MR because of claustrophobia. T_1-weighted axial MRI demonstrates a fresh thrombus within the arterial wall after dissection while MRA shows tapering of the internal carotid artery stump.

In those with premature atherosclerosis who do not possess the usual risk factors, homocystinuria should be excluded. Homozygotes, who have a marfanoid habitus, can be identified by elevated blood/urine homocystine levels and a positive nitroprusside test while heterozygotes, who have a lower risk of atherosclerosis, may require a methionine loading test to demonstrate the metabolic defect.

In a normotensive person with a normal ipsilateral carotid artery, a cardiac cause should be excluded using echocardiography. However, in the absence of clinical signs, transthoracic echocardiography has a low diagnostic yield. It can demonstrate ventricular and atrial thrombi, valvular vegetations and large atrial septal defects, but can miss small significant lesions. Transoesophageal echocardiography is a semi-invasive technique which more clearly visualizes left atrial appendage thrombi and valvular vegetations.

A cardiac source of emboli is identified in 20–30% of cases. Commonest causes are prosthetic heart valves, rheumatic valvular disease, infective endocarditis, dilated cardiomyopathy and ischaemic dyskinetic segments. Other findings, e.g. atrial septal aneurysm, patent foramen ovale and mitral valve prolapse are of debatable significance.

Prothrombotic states

When embolism from extracranial or cardiac sources has been excluded, attention should focus on exclusion of prothrombotic conditions. While these are rare, they are increasingly recognized as a cause of stroke in young people. Furthermore, lifelong anticoagulation is indicated and, therefore, haematological screening is essential.

Primary abnormalities of the coagulation and fibrinolytic system are associated with venous and, to a lesser extent, arterial thrombosis. Inherited thrombophilias (deficiencies of protein C, S, antithrombin) are common, but symptomatic deficiencies are rare.

Lupus anticoagulant and anticardiolipin antibodies are present in 50% of patients with lupus and other autoimmune disease. They are also found in patients with recurrent venous and arterial thrombosis, spontaneous abortion and livedo reticularis, where their presence is an independent risk factor for cerebral infarction.

Intracranial vasculitis

This would be an unusual cause of a stroke in someone who has otherwise been well. However, CNS vasculitis can occur as an isolated phenomenon or as the presenting feature of a systemic necrotizing vasculitis. Other causes of arteritis include autoimmune disease, certain infections or neoplastic conditions, and drugs. Even in the absence of systemic clues, a thorough immunological screen is justifiable in any young person presenting with a stroke.

Isolated CNS angiitis is a very rare condition, which usually presents with an encephalopathy, but can cause an acute stroke. There are no symptoms outwith the CNS, no peripheral markers and neurological tests (CSF, EEG, MRI) reveal non-specific findings only. Angiography demonstrates multiple segmental narrowing in small/medium-sized vessels in 50% of cases but definitive diagnosis requires leptomeningeal/cerebral biopsy. This is only justifiable in the presence of clinical deterioration with negative angiography, when it should be performed because treatment (steroids plus cyclophosphamide) may be curative.

Miscellaneous causes

Migraine

Case-control studies reveal an increased susceptibility to stroke in young women with migraine, especially those who smoke. Whether the oral contraceptive pill is an additional independent risk factor is not known. However, in the majority of women with migraine who have a stroke, migraine is not the cause. Furthermore, carotid dissection can mimic migraine resulting in misdiagnosis of the cause of the stroke. Therefore, very strict requirements for the diagnosis of 'migrainous stroke' have evolved. These are: an ischaemic event developing in someone who has migraine with aura; the provoking attack should be identical to previous attacks; the neurological deficit should persist for longer than 7 days; and other causes must be excluded.

Drug abuse

In recent series, drug abuse is reported to be a leading cause of stroke in young people. Cerebral infarction occurs with abuse of heroin, cocaine, amphetamines and over-the-counter sympathomimetic compounds. The commonest mechanism is obliterative arteritis caused by immune complex deposition consequent upon prolonged challenge with foreign antigen. Stroke usually occurs between 6 and 24 hours after drug administration.

Genetics

A recently identified, single-gene disorder, cerebral autosomal dominant arteriopathy with subcortical infarcts and leucoencephalopathy (CADASIL), has been localized to chromosome 19. This condition typically presents with stroke or TIA followed by a progressive decline with pseudobulbar palsy and dementia. MRI reveals multiple small infarcts in deep white matter. Other inherited conditions which predispose to stroke include mitochondrial disease (MELAS), while some connective tissue disorders cause cervical artery dissection.

Conclusion

In a young person, a diagnosis of stroke *per se* is insufficient. These individuals should be investigated in a specialist centre to establish the aetiology. Advances in MR technology (arterial dissection) and understanding of haematology/immunology (prothrombotic states) permit identification of hitherto underdiagnosed or unrecognized conditions. Precise diagnoses have implications for secondary prevention and prognosis.

References

Martin PJ, Enevoldson TP, Humphrey PRD. Causes of ischaemic stroke in the young. *Postgrad Med J* 1997, **73**, 8–16.

Commonly performed investigations in young stroke patients

General	Specific
• Full blood count	• Clotting profile
• Erythrocyte sedimentation rate	• Proteins C & S, antithrombin III
• Biochemistry screen	• Haemoglobin electrophoresis
• Glucose	• Lupus anticoagulant
• Cholesterol and triglycerides	• Anticardiolipin antibodies
• Electrocardiogram	• Antinuclear antibodies and dsDNA antibodies
• Chest X-ray	• VDRL/TPHA
• CT brain scan	• HIV
	• Urine drug screen
	• Urine homocysteine/nitroprusside test
	• Methionine loading test
	• Muscle biopsy
	• DNA analysis
	• Cerebrospinal fluid analysis
	• Transthoracic echocardiography
	• Transoesophageal echocardiography
	• Carotid/vertebral artery ultrasound
	• MRI scan (brain and neck)
	• MRA intra- and extracranial arteries
	• Intra-arterial carotid/vertebral angiography
	• Leptomeningeal and brain biopsy

Index